Late Babies

Late Babies

Having a baby after 35

SANDRA McLEAN

BANTAM
SYDNEY • AUCKLAND • TORONTO • NEW YORK • LONDON

LATE BABIES
A BANTAM BOOK

First published in Australia and New Zealand in 2004
by Bantam

National Library of Australia
Cataloguing-in-Publication Entry

McLean, Sandra.
  Late babies: having a baby after 35

  Bibliography.
  ISBN 1 86325 446 3.

  1. Mothers – Australia – Interviews. 2. Pregnancy in
  middle age – Australia. 3. Childbirth in middle age –
  Australia. I. Title

306.87430994

Transworld Publishers,
a division of Random House Australia Pty Ltd
20 Alfred Street, Milsons Point, NSW 2061
http://www.randomhouse.com.au

Random House New Zealand Limited
18 Poland Road, Glenfield, Auckland

Transworld Publishers,
a division of The Random House Group Ltd
61-63 Uxbridge Road, Ealing, London W5 5SA

Random House Inc
1745 Broadway, New York, New York 10036

Edited by Amanda O'Connell
Cover photo by Gandee Vasan/Getty Images
Typeset in 13/17.5 pt Garamond 3 by Midland Typesetters, Maryborough, Victoria
Printed and bound by Griffin Press, Netley, South Australia

10 9 8 7 6 5 4 3 2 1

To my parents, Ron and Judy McLean, who let me live my life, and my husband, Phil Brown, and son, Hamish, who changed my life.

Contents

Introduction

I WAS 38 BEFORE I held a newborn baby. When I did, it happened to be mine, a boy my husband and I named Hamish. We were glad he was a boy because we hadn't been able to agree on any female names. In fact, we had found it hard to concentrate on the whole experience of having a baby. Even when I found out I was pregnant in October 1999, it was difficult to focus on the concept that in nine months, if all went well, Phil and I would be holding a baby – our baby. Reality set in quickly, however, after Hamish was born in July 2000.

Looking back, I blame my baby blur on the fact my husband, Phil Brown, and I were busy being globetrotting professionals. We were (and still are) journalists who preferred inner-city life and all the convenience that goes with this. We get the sweats if we have to visit someone who lives further than ten kilometres from the CBD. We were better skilled at snaring the best seats in the coolest cafés than deciding which colour to paint the nursery or which pram to buy our precious offspring.

We hadn't spent our married life focused on having babies – quite the opposite. In the eight years we were married before Hamish was born, we concentrated on work, holidays, surfing and satisfying our personal needs. Looking back we were very self-indulgent and wasted a heck of a lot of time. I suppose, too, like many women who have had babies later in life, I wondered why I waited so long to have a child.

I realise now that we were living in a cocoon, closeted from the ways of most of the world, or at least that part of the world involved in child-rearing. I can remember going to Noosa, the Queensland Sunshine Coast holiday haven, after Hamish was born and being amazed at how many other people were pushing newborns around in designer prams or balancing a cappuccino in one hand and a toddler in the other. Had it always been this way, I wondered out loud to Phil, or had my pre-parental existence been so self-obsessed that I had simply failed to notice? This was a shock to me as I had always considered myself alert to my surroundings. Obviously, I hadn't been paying attention.

In the same way, when Hamish was born I failed to notice the gravity of my achievement: first, that at the ripe old age of 38 I was lucky to have conceived; secondly, I had given birth to a healthy child; and thirdly, I had survived the experience with my health and sanity intact. Also, in having a child this late in life I was unwittingly part of the strengthening trend in Australia and most of the Western world for women to delay childbirth.

I had become one of those statistics recorded by the Australian Bureau of Statistics showing that 1 in 10 Australian women are having their first baby when they are aged 35 years or older. By the start of the twenty-first century, 1 in 2 births were to women in this age group. This compares to just under 1 in 4 in 1979.

This trend is happening in the face of biological fact. Many women who have delayed childbirth until their late thirties or early forties find out – too late – that they cannot get pregnant. Sometimes this can be because of infertility problems experienced by their partner. However, one of the key problems with older women wanting to get pregnant is age-related infertility. Sadly, this can be a biological fact of life that even advanced reproductive medicine cannot change. Fertility treatment such as in-vitro fertilisation (IVF) cannot yet move back the hands of the biological clock.

Of course, reproductive medicine is constantly striving to find ways to try to give women precious extra time. Any new discoveries will give hope to many women but it could be years before any research being carried out today has pragmatic outcomes. In the meantime, women are still faced with the scenario of trying to fit it all in – the career, the relationship and the family – before it is too late.

In writing this book, I spoke to mothers of late babies whose stories sounded very similar to mine. Some had only realised retrospectively their great good luck in conceiving and carrying their baby to term. Others had experienced the heartbreak of miscarriage, which brought them face to face with fertility's version of the glass ceiling. Then there were others who broke through this glass ceiling, either with the help of fertility treatment such as IVF or by what they often refer to as a 'miracle' natural conception.

I wanted to find out from them the real story behind a modern-day phenomenon: the Western trend to delaying motherhood. Why had these women waited to have children? Was it because of career, lifestyle, lack of a good partner or a combination of all of these? Each of their stories is a mini-memoir which I hope will give some insight into the complexities of older motherhood as well as communicating the joy in having that hard-won, much-loved late baby.

Sandra McLean

June 2004

Maggie Alderson
author and fashion columnist

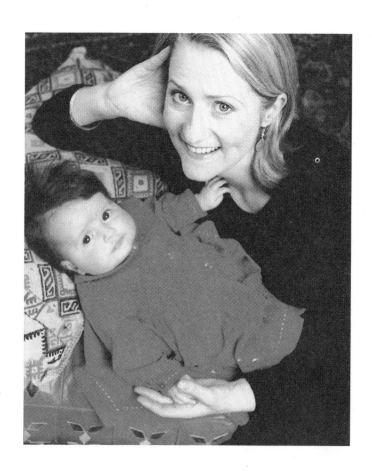

'If you ask me why I left it so late to have a baby, I say now that it is the cumulative effect of decisions — it is something that you learn as you get older. Every decision you make adds up to your future. It is also about circumstances and choices.'

MOST OF US HAVE heard the classic story of finally finding Mr Right: the moment a woman gives up in despair and switches off the male-seeking radar, ding-dong, he arrives on her doorstep. It's uncanny, really.

Maggie Alderson, one of Australia's favourite fashion columnists and the author of two best-selling novels, uses this Mr Right analogy to try to explain the emotions she experienced when, at 42, she discovered — in the loo of her London literary agent — that she was pregnant.

She was elated and a little surprised. After all, Maggie had given up on falling pregnant. Instead of looking for a man, Maggie, since her late thirties, had been looking for ways to have a child. She'd already found her Mr Right, Popi Popovic, a retired professional soccer player, and for four years they had been trying to conceive, with no success.

This had been a desperate time, rife with conflicting emotions and disappointments as Maggie tried to stem a rising tide of grief and unhappiness because of her inability to conceive. She later described this feeling as a 'gnawing pain' inside her.

After years of working hard at a career that took her to the top in magazines in both the United Kingdom and Australia, Maggie, perhaps like many other women of her generation, had not paid any particular attention to having children. She always thought she could have them when she wanted, that is, when the right man came along and when there was a suitable time in her career to take a mummy break. But Maggie was to learn – almost too late – that female fertility is finite. The world may be full of infinite career opportunities and fashion seasons, but there is a limit to a woman's fecundity.

Even so, this doesn't deter a woman who is determined to have a child. So Maggie flirted with Ayurvedic medicine, a traditional holistic system developed in India, in an attempt to boost her fertility. She had acupuncture treatment. Together, she and Popi contemplated assisted reproductive technology (ART) like in-vitro fertilisation (IVF); however they changed their minds at the last minute.

In desperation, Maggie even considered adoption, even though she knew her husband did not want to take this route. Just as she was secretly devising tactics for a pro-adoption campaign, aimed at changing Popi's mind, Maggie fell pregnant naturally. That pro-adoption slogan was no longer needed.

It was a miracle for me to fall pregnant. That's the way I felt. It was definitely a miracle. An extraordinary miracle. My family was so happy for me when they found out – although they had done their best to hide it, they were very sad I had not had children. I'm one of four children and all my siblings have children. I loved being an auntie but I knew my family felt a little sad for me that I had never had kids. So when I announced I was pregnant their happiness was lovely.

On 18 July 2002, Maggie gave birth to Peggy, becoming a first-time mum two weeks before her forty-third birthday. While I am interviewing Maggie, her little 'miracle' is sleeping. Ordinarily, this would be a chance for Maggie to make the most of some valuable time to write. She is putting the final touches to the manuscript for her third novel, due out in 2004. Of course Maggie works as a journalist and columnist as well. She has twenty-six years' experience in the media and is an internationally regarded fashion writer, whose quirky, opinionated and highly personal 'Style Notes' column appears weekly in the *Age* and *Sydney Morning Herald* newspapers in Australia. She also writes for numerous publications in the United Kingdom and the United States.

Maggie's career has taken her around the world countless times. She's mingled with the rich and glamorous. Parties, oh yes, there have been many of those. And the invitations are still arriving in her letterbox, but these days the fashion world has to party without Maggie.

Since Peggy was born, her commitment to work and to being a mum has proved more important than parties. Not that Maggie minds the change of pace in her life.

Sometimes I do get invited to something and I think wistfully about going out, but now I can't. I look at Peggy's little face and it earths me. It brings me down to the real things that matter in life. Earlier today I had her standing at the kitchen sink and she was playing with the washing-up brush — she was so happy just to do that.

We are constantly searching in our life for the big thrill — for some people it might be bungee jumping. For me it might be getting a new Prada handbag. But we are surrounded by the greatest miracle of all and that is children. I really feel we have lost touch with that because in olden times it was hard to live a life without contact with children or babies. Now you can live a life that is barren of children. I did for a long time. When I was living in Sydney before Peggy was born most of my friends were gay or single — none of us had kids. I would go for weeks without some kind of interaction with a child. I think that is wrong.

Anyone who has read Maggie's fashion journalism might be amazed to hear her revel unabashedly in life's simple things. After all, up until Peggy's birth, Maggie's world wasn't exactly focused on the kitchen sink. She has long been associated with the fashion scene after making her first foray into journalism when she started her own punk rock fanzine in 1977. She went on to work in key roles on glossy magazines such as *Elle*, where she was editor-in-chief, in the United Kingdom and *Cleo* in Australia as well as on several English newspapers, including the *Evening Standard*. Her work at the *Evening Standard* won her the British Society of Magazine Editors 'Editor of the Year' award in 1989. She moved to Sydney in 1993 to edit the stylish *Mode* magazine, before moving to the *Sydney Morning Herald* as a senior writer, starting the 'Style Notes' column six years ago.

At a glance, fashion doesn't appear to be the kind of world which dwells for too long on the nitty-gritty of motherhood. Pulped pumpkin and dirty nappies clash badly with the catwalks of Milan. Maggie says, however, that fashion is a relatively mummy-friendly business. After all, much of the fashion world is made up of women, and many of them are mums.

It's really funny at the fashion shows — one season I see bumps and then the woman is gone for a season and then next time she is back showing her baby photos! It is hard for me being away from Peggy for two weeks twice a year doing the shows, but it has to be done. I tell myself that at least she sees a lot of me in my normal working day. Popi normally takes her to stay with his parents while I am at the shows, so at least I know she is being looked after by the best possible people and thoroughly spoiled, too.

There's also the rising tide of haute couture for infants to consider, although according to Maggie, keeping one's offspring fashionably dressed can be a challenge — even if model mums such as Elle Macpherson and Kate Moss seem to carry it off with aplomb. New mum Maggie canvassed the contradiction that is elegance and babywear in one of her 'Style Notes' columns soon after Peggy was born, in which she acknowledged that high fashion and infants rarely make a good mix.

Another hurdle between me and a beautifully turned out baby is the washing. Babies vomit a lot and do horrible things with bananas. So anything that has to be hand-washed or ironed generally gets besmirched immediately and then sits at the bottom of the laundry bin or ironing mountain until the child has started school. Which is why you can get such bargains at baby clothes sales.

The flippant tone is classic Alderson, and even when she recounts her own story of how she almost didn't become a mother there is amusement in her voice. It's as if she still can't believe her good fortune at becoming a mum.

Yes, she says, it is true that she listened to a Sydney Gay and Lesbian Mardi Gras compilation CD during a long and painful labour before giving birth to Peggy.

If I sucked down enough gas and air I felt quite out of it and had a great little disco dance. It took my mind off 30 hours of labour pains without any other pain relief. I also had Chopin but the disco music was much better.

Maggie asks me if I've seen a recent newspaper story about birth plans that went wrong. It mentioned a woman who was so fed up with the way her labour had gone so badly *not* according to plan that she set fire to her carefully calculated birth notes.

That was me. I had about six copies of the birth plan, which I took to the hospital with me. When I took one out to show the midwife she just rolled her eyes as if to say, 'Not another one.' I wanted to have a water birth but I couldn't get into the water birthing room at the hospital when I needed to. After 30 hours of labour, with no pain relief, except gas, with a cervix completely undilated, I ceremonially tore up the birth plan.

Her birth plan in shreds, Maggie eventually gave birth to Peggy after an emergency Caesarean and, in the end, with her two girlfriends and husband, Popi, close at hand, that was all that mattered. She may joke now about her long and difficult labour, tossing caustic comments at the natural birth 'coven' and how she felt 'sucked in' by their insistence on a drug-free labour. However, underneath it all there is a sense of relief that she managed to cheat the biological clock and fall pregnant naturally at 42, then maintain the pregnancy and have a healthy baby girl.

Maggie says she never made a conscious decision to delay having a baby. It was just that by the time she reached her late thirties she had simply not got around to it. The demands of her busy life had diverted the path to motherhood.

If you ask me why I left it so late to have a baby, I say now that it is the cumulative effect of decisions – it is something that you learn as you get older. Every decision you make adds up to your future. It is also about circumstances and choices.

The man I chose to be with for twelve years did not want to have children and they were my prime reproductive years. I was also very career-orientated. I chose to get a swanky new job instead of staying with a newspaper that had really good maternity leave. I'd had a secure job and at that point my boyfriend of the time was wavering about being a parent. I was 28. Instead of staying and having a family, I decided to get a new high-pressure job. They were my decisions.

Also, there was my pathetic ignorance of how conception worked.

Even though I am a doctor's daughter, I did not really

understand female fertility. I could write a thesis on contraception, but I understood very little about conception.

Maggie was to receive a crash course on fertility and conception when a girlfriend showed her a chart that had been given to her by her gynaecologist. The chart indicated that a woman's fertility starts to droop at 34 or 35, then seriously sags at 37, before flopping badly in her early forties and then virtually disappearing in her mid-forties.

I was stunned. The chart showed there was this cliff at 37 when your fertility dropped away. I saw this chart just before my thirty-eighth birthday. It was one of the most awful moments of my life. I had not realised that the female reproductive system closes down quite suddenly. I thought it was a gradual slide.

After seeing the graph, Maggie decided she needed to have a serious talk with Popi. They had been together for several years and had talked about having children. He had wanted to wait a bit longer so they could enjoy their life together and then think about it in a few years time.

He (Popi) couldn't believe his ears when I told him (about female fertility). Like everyone else he said to me, 'What about Cherie Blair? What about Madonna?'

True, Cherie Blair, wife of the British prime minister, Tony Blair, had given birth at 45 to her fourth child, Leo. But any fertility expert will tell you this is definitely not the norm. The media, however, tends to emphasise these cases, giving glowing reports of celebrity older mums like Cherie and the pop star Madonna. However we are not privy to the full circumstances of their pregnancies or any difficulties they may have had falling pregnant. These facts tend to be kept private by celebrities, and that's their prerogative. Even so, reading about their babies can create a false sense of security in other women. It's understandable they may think, heck, if Madonna can have her first child at 38, then why can't I? Never mind that both Madonna and Cherie Blair are better placed financially than most regular late-in-life mums or that even hi-tech reproductive science sometimes cannot improve the diminishing fertility of a woman in her mid to late forties.

Getting pregnant is a gamble at any stage in a woman's life – out of one hundred couples under the age of 35 trying to conceive, only twenty will be successful in any given month and of those twenty, three will miscarry.[1] These odds get tougher as the woman ages. According to clinical estimates, once a woman reaches her early forties she has only a 5 per cent chance of getting pregnant using her own eggs.

As a result, women like Cherie Blair and Maggie Alderson are not the statistical norm. As Maggie says: 'Cherie Blair is a statistical freak. And now so am I.'

When Maggie saw the gynaecologist's chart she decided she could no longer be indecisive about motherhood. She had to take affirmative action. So she and Popi started trying to conceive. Maggie tried to give herself the best chance of falling pregnant by keeping track of when she was ovulating, using the traditional method of taking her temperature. She also had acupuncture treatment and tried Ayurvedic medicine. Nothing worked. And Ayurvedic therapy was very undignified.

You reach a point where you say that is enough bollocks. The Ayurvedic medicine was the end of bollocks for me. The doctor gave me packets of powder that he wanted me to put on my fanny. I thought, this is just ridiculous. We tried for a year taking temperatures and trying to have sex according to the ovulation chart, but I didn't fall pregnant.

That is when our gynaecologist said we needed to do an investigation — to see if there was any medical reason, apart from my age, to explain why I couldn't fall pregnant. When nothing was found, that was when we started to go down the IVF path.

Maggie says she wasn't keen on having fertility treatment. Her attitude had been influenced by the experiences of women she knew who were having IVF and had failed to fall pregnant. The drugs that are part of the IVF treatment had taken a terrible toll on one friend in particular.

I was getting these emails from one friend every day through her IVF treatment; she went bonkers and she didn't get pregnant. And it cost her a fortune. Then, what really finished it off for me were the odds. I like horseracing and I looked at the odds and they said you had a 20 per cent chance of success. Well, that is five to one, which are really crap odds. That is an 80 per cent chance of failure. I don't mind buying a lottery ticket with those odds but I started to feel as though I was not prepared to go through that incredible hormonal stress.

Then in her early forties, Maggie was forced to consider the very real possibility that she might not have children. She knew that she wanted a child but she also knew that she wanted to feel comfortable with her conscience. Maggie decided it was time to live with those decisions that had led her headlong down a successful career path and into relationships where children were not a priority. After years of not really making any decisions about having children of her own, she acted.

The time was nearing for Maggie to start her first cycle of IVF. She decided she didn't want to go through with it. Popi, who is two years older than Maggie, accepted her decision.

He was really relieved. He was incredibly supportive. I think he was more fifty-fifty about having a child than me. He would have been equally happy to have a really nice life without a child. He sympathised with me because he knew that, as a woman, I had this inner gnawing pain to have a child.

But I had begun to think about it. Morally, I felt as if I could not go through IVF. There are certain decisions that I had made in my life that had brought me to this point. And I had to take responsibility for those decisions.

So at that point I decided I was not going to have a baby and I would have to accept that. I'd had a pretty amazing life, travelled the world and I thought I would just carry on having lots of adventures and lead a different life without children. The time comes when you have to take responsibility for those decisions and realise that you can't have everything.

In Maggie's mind she had made a decision – but her heart wasn't in it. She recalls how, after pulling out of the IVF treatment, she went to Vietnam with a friend who was adopting a baby. It felt like a good idea, considering Maggie still wanted a child. However, Popi did not agree with adoption.

He was absolutely against adoption. I don't know why he was against it but he respected my wishes and I had to respect his and it was all part of that thing that not everybody has kids. I thought I could have another life. I have nieces and nephews and I thought I could be their mad aunt.

But just as Maggie had started trying to come to terms with being childless and to focus instead on her burgeoning career as a writer of fiction, life dealt her a surprise. Six weeks after her visit to Vietnam, Maggie missed a period. Then aged 42, she thought it was the start of menopause.

I was driving with my mum and asked her, 'What age did you start menopause?' She gave me a funny look and asked why. I told her that I had missed my period and she said, 'You'd better have a pregnancy test.'

I found out I was pregnant in the loo of my agent's office in London. I'd just bought a pregnancy testing kit from the chemist at Piccadilly Circus and couldn't wait another second before trying it! Oh, the beauty of those little blue lines.

This pregnancy wasn't supposed to happen. But it did. Maggie still searches for an explanation. She ponders the elements in her life during the autumn of 2001 that might have made a difference to her fertility. Let's see, she was living a relatively healthy life at the time, eating well and not drinking a lot of alcohol. She had started working from home and she was feeling relaxed and happy. She had been to Vietnam where she had been with babies in the orphanage.

*I don't know if any of these things made a difference . . . how
do you know? All I know is that I had a wonderful pregnancy.
I absolutely loved every minute of it.*

Peggy's birth was a new beginning for Maggie – and
changed everything. Maggie tells how friends had described
how having a new baby rearranged everything, from sleep
patterns to furniture. 'It changes your life beyond recognition,'
Maggie says.

Peggy was three weeks old when Maggie wrote her first piece
of journalism as a new mother. Finding some sort of equilibrium
between work and baby was difficult at first. Part of the problem
is the very nature of journalism and writing. The work varies
from day to day. Sometimes weekends have to be worked. Other
times, deadlines demand work be done late into the night. As
well as her journalism which included her 'Style Notes' column
and magazine pieces, Maggie was working on a novel, following the success of her previous two novels, *Pants on Fire* and *Mad
About the Boy*. At the time of our interview, her third book was
six months behind schedule. 'Guess why,' Maggie laughs.

Finding that middle ground between work and baby is a
challenge for any new mother. Throw in a desire for some time
of your own and the need to nourish an adult relationship with
your partner and things start to get really complicated.
Maggie's situation after Peggy's birth was coloured by the fact
that she was not only a first-time mother, but also an older
mother.

Peggy is a special baby, the child that Maggie thought she
would never have. Consequently, she put on hold any plans to
put Peggy in child care. She and Popi, whom Maggie married

in January 2002, have split the care and make use of various kinds of home help, including a nanny who looks after Peggy two days a week. Maggie often works at night, writing into the early hours of the morning.

The rest of the time we split it, but also consciously make time to spend with her together, which I think is really important too. It involves more sacrifice (I could be working/sleeping/having a pedicure), but I am prepared to make sacrifices while she is little. It is too precious.

I can't say it has been easy but I think all parents just muddle along as best they can. We could have packed her off to day care, but I just didn't want to. I waited so long for this baby I want to see as much of her as I can, even if it is just stopping for a chat when I go downstairs to make a cup of tea.

Popi has been absolutely amazing about doing all the night wake-up stuff so I can sleep as I need my brain for work. He is the most amazing father and I think Peggy is a very lucky girl to see so much of him.

I would have finished my book a year ago, but with Peggy I have found that there is a point where I just don't want to be away from her. She was such a miracle child. It is possible that if I was younger and maybe had a chance of having more children I would have been a little bit more easygoing about her care. However because it is likely that she is the only child I will have I didn't want to miss out on too much time with her.

Being an older mum is a challenge and Maggie says that she often feels tired when her sleep is broken by her toddler's cry. She can also feel frustrated when she can't sit down to write because her child's demands on her time are stronger. However, she believes that she worries less than she might about the restrictions having a baby has put on her life because she has done so much already. Besides, she says, her nightclubbing days were over by the time Peggy came along.

At 45, Maggie is acutely aware that she will be in her sixties by the time Peggy is in her twenties. Being older also means she can't rely on her parents to babysit Peggy. Even so there is the joy in seeing her mother, who is in her eighties, spend time with Peggy. (Maggie's father died twenty years ago.) Being in her mid-forties also makes Maggie aware that she will most probably not have another child. Of course, she has thought about it.

I would love to have another child to provide a sibling for Peggy's sake. I feel quite guilty about that. I grew up in a big family and we had so much fun. I would love her to have a sibling – I don't want her to be a self-centred child. Then again, some of the most interesting people I know are only children.

But is it too much to ask for two miracles in one life? Maggie knows that at 45 her chances of a natural conception are even smaller than they were three years ago when Peggy was conceived. The risks of miscarriage are greater and the chances are higher of chromosomal abnormality in the foetus. Besides, Maggie feels that she shouldn't push her luck.

I have talked about this to other women who are older and have had children and we tend to feel that we are so incredibly lucky to have a healthy baby at our age. The odds to do what we have done already sound terrifying. So, part of me thinks I don't want to risk it (having another child).

Also, something in Maggie rejects that twenty-first century mantra: 'I want it no matter what.' This may be fine if we're talking about the latest Prada handbag, but is it sustainable when the same desire is directed at children?

I don't think you can really have it all. Also, I don't think that you can truly engineer life. Conception is the great mystery of life and I just wonder how much man should be interfering with it. For younger women who are trying to get pregnant, I can see the benefits of IVF, but for older women, who have made certain choices in their lives, I have a certain discomfort with that. It is as if we want it all – we want career, freedom, travel and fun, and we want the baby as well, please. I know what it feels like to want to have that child. And I really feel that I have been lucky in that I have been able to have a child late in life – but I was a fluke and don't take me as an example.

Peggy was a miracle. I would say to young women: Really understand your reproductive system and search into your soul and try and know yourself. Do you really want to have children? How important is it to you? Weigh it up with your career and ask yourself which is more important. If children are more important, then you ought to get on with it, because later on you might not have a choice.

Juanita Phillips

journalist and ABC newsreader

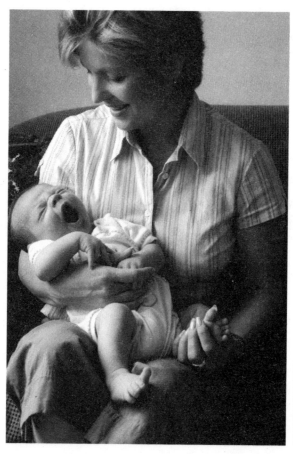

HELEN COETZEE

'Just about every woman wants to have a child, and given the right circumstances – finding a good man who wants to have children with you – they will.'

MANY WOMEN WHO talk about having a baby later in life use the word 'lucky' to describe their situation. For these women in their late thirties or early forties, giving birth to a healthy child is akin to winning the lottery. They simply can't believe their luck.

But having a baby late in life is not only about luck, it is also a salient lesson in the way life can suddenly veer into unknown terrain.

These were my thoughts on the plane back to Brisbane after I interviewed Juanita Phillips, national broadcaster ABC-TV's prime-time newsreader – and new mother at 40. We had spent the afternoon at her mother-in-law's house in Sydney's northern suburbs, Juanita happy to sit on the couch breastfeeding her newborn son, Marcus. Her husband of seven months, Mario Milostic, a graphic designer, was at work. His mother, Marija, alternated between making us coffee and helping out with Marcus. We talked about the miracle of birth, the sudden responsibility of motherhood and the often farcical times faced by new parents who, despite their mature age and apparent skill in the workplace, often have little idea what to do with a newborn baby.

Juanita also talked about how lucky she was to have Marcus. She had turned 40 only days before he was born late in 2003, and his birth was a true gift, as Juanita had spent most of her late thirties believing her desire to become a mother would never be fulfilled.

I feel as if I just got through the door before it shut. I do feel lucky in meeting Mario and the way it all happened to me, getting married and getting pregnant. When I was 37 or 38 I was deeply sad about missing out on being a mother because I really wanted to have a child and a family.

They say you always remember things for a reason and I remember I was at a television party in London and I was talking to this woman who was some high-flying banker and at one point she said, 'I've got to get going as I've got to get my babies to bed.' She was obviously in her early forties and my ears pricked up and I said, 'Oh, you have young children?' She said yes, she'd had them really quickly and that she was into her career, thought she'd missed out, then, at 38, she met her future husband on a date and six months later they got married and immediately had two kids. I always remember then thinking that maybe I can still do it, maybe it can still happen and it sort of happened that way for me.

Juanita's comments stayed in my mind as they echoed what I had already heard from many mothers of late babies who had also given up on having children. They, too, realised that you never know how life can change.

Before our interview, the last time I had seen Juanita was at least three years before in the offices of the *Courier-Mail*, the Brisbane newspaper where I work as a feature writer and where Juanita had started in journalism in 1982. Then on holiday from her high-profile job as London anchor for the cable news channel CNN, Juanita was the local girl made good. She was a success on the newspaper just about from the day she started until the day she left to become a reporter and newsreader for Channel 10 in Brisbane.

With her gamine beauty, crisp diction and strong background in journalism, Juanita easily made the crossover from print to television. Her star continued to rise after leaving Ten to join the subscriber television news channel Sky News in Sydney, where she stayed for two years before going to London. There, after almost giving up after weeks of disappointments, she managed to break into international newsreading, first getting a job with BBC World and then snaring a key role with the huge American cable channel CNN. In London, she continued writing a series of children's books, called *The Newspaper Kids*, first published in 1996.

Juanita had come back to Brisbane to visit her family and old friends. Never haughty with her success, she was happy to be away from the high-pressure world of 24-hour international television news. We talked about work and living in London, where she had also briefly been a part-owner of a café.

Babies were not mentioned. And why would they be?

Juanita was a success in her chosen profession, having been head-hunted by CNN after proving her worth at BBC World where she calmly reported on the death of Diana, Princess of Wales, in 1997, only two days into her job with the broad-caster. During her time with CNN she had refused to be desk bound, reporting on the violent anti-globalisation riots in Prague in 2000 and covering the unpredictable Kosovo crisis. With a London flat and a high-profile job, Juanita, her passport in her handbag in case of emergency, was living the dream of many a young female television journalist.

And then, almost five years into her time in the United Kingdom and only a few years after I had seen her in Brisbane, she quit the so-called dream job. Juanita packed her bags, cleared out her London apartment and flew back to Australia. She was 38. In May 2002, Juanita started reading the weekend news for the ABC, then, in January 2003, joined Tony Eastley to read the 7pm news for the national broadcaster.

Many of Juanita's colleagues couldn't believe she had left CNN in London to work for the ABC in Sydney. The cynical observer might have described it as career suicide. So what caused this seismic change in Juanita's life? It would be trite to say that she left her job to have a baby. At that point, Juanita didn't even have a boyfriend. And her dedication to the job seemed to indicate that motherhood was never more than a blip on her personal radar.

However, those close to Juanita knew differently. She told me that during her thirties, when she was outwardly the very image of success, privately she was disappointed by her failure to have a baby.

During those years in London she had thought an awful lot

about having a child. Her desire for a family was connected to a deep yearning for something more in her life than workaday success. In particular, she wanted a strong, loving relationship with a man which would produce children. These feelings intensified as she moved into her late thirties and became aware of her diminishing fertility. Her fortieth birthday was looming. Juanita had known many deadlines in her life, but this one was personal.

Her yearning for a child was a late development – in her twenties Juanita had been happy to pursue her career and adventure.

I was much more work-focused because that was when for the first time a lot of women were not getting married in their twenties and then having kids in their thirties. So when I was in my twenties I didn't give having children much thought. I travelled a lot, did the whole backpacking thing and had a lot of fun. It was only in my early thirties I wanted to have kids. I left it this late for a whole lot of reasons, but one big reason was that I had a series of relationships and I did not meet men who wanted to have children and get married. That was a real issue and so in the absence of that I pursued my career and did very well. Then it just became a career thing, in that I was working long hours and doing well at my job. At that stage having children was something that was pushed to the back of my mind. From the age of 37 I accepted that I was not going to have children and I thought that was fine, I have missed the boat. I had made choices to pursue my career and this is the consequence of that. It took me a few years to come to terms with it. There was a period in my thirties when I was unhappy because I was thinking, 'Did I make a mistake?'

Then I came to a nice space where I realised I had made my choices. When I look back at that time now I wouldn't swap it. I am really pleased that I had those years of travelling and being completely selfish and doing what I wanted. I am so happy now that I have this very ordinary life. I never go out and I am not interested in clothes and eating out in restaurants — not like I used to be. I am pleased I did all of that because I know that it is nice to do and have but it is ultimately empty.

I think that is why I had such a terrific pregnancy. There was nothing left in my professional life that I wanted to do. I have written children's books, worked for newspapers and CNN and the BBC and travelled for a few years as a backpacker. There is nothing left that I really want to do except spend time with my husband and baby and potter around the house. If I had a child before I went to London maybe I would have always thought to myself: 'Could I have gone further?'

By her late thirties Juanita had gone a long way, but her desire for something more in life than work gained the upper hand after the September 11, 2001 terrorist attacks on the World Trade Center in New York and the Pentagon in Washington, DC. She told me that the attacks rocked her out of her complacency, causing her to quit her top-level job at CNN.

It was a very odd time in London, very tense. No one would travel on public transport and it was a strange time at CNN, too, because as it was an American network it was considered a target for terrorists. There was a lot of tension and stress and I just wanted to come home. That time in London, including those five years at CNN, was hard. CNN is a tough company – they are good to you but you have to give them your pound of flesh. It was a hard job and I realised that I wanted a life where family was more important and where I had time to see my friends and family and have some time for myself.

Juanita also realised that one of the reasons she had done so well at CNN was that as a single woman without children she was always available to work.

It wasn't so much the long hours that got to me at CNN – it was the shocking shifts. Being an international broadcaster there is no nine-to-five culture. I was always doing breakfast so I had to start work at two in the morning, five days a week. With the BBC I did some midnight to 8am shifts. It was a shock and I can still remember realising that the reason I had done so well at CNN was that I was available – I was single and I had no children. I was available to do unsocial hours. If someone called in sick, then they called me. If they needed someone to jump on a train to Paris I could do that as I always had my passport with me. I had no personal responsibilities and it became clear to me that is why married women with children tend to disappear off the radar – they are not available to do the hours that corporate life or this busy kind of media life requires you to do.

Once her decision was made, Juanita moved quickly and was back in Sydney by early 2002. She had been born in Sydney but grew up in Brisbane, so the city was a little strange to her. At least the job at the ABC was familiar. Only a few months after starting at the national broadcaster, Juanita's life was about to be turned upside down.

She had met Mario in a Sydney café. They went on a few dates and seven weeks into their romance Mario proposed to Juanita over a picnic at Pearl Beach on the New South Wales Central Coast.

It happened really quickly for us. When we met I had no expectations – by that point I could have given up on having children and accepted that these days it is hard to find a man who wants to commit to a relationship and a family.

All I hoped for at that point was that I could meet a lifelong partner and have a good relationship. I had dropped the idea that children were essential to my happiness, through sheer necessity – I didn't want to live the rest of my life wishing for something I didn't have.

So when Mario and I got together I had no expectations about the relationship. I just thought he was a great guy. I was simply enjoying our relationship day to day. In fact when Mario proposed, I was so shocked. I was literally speechless. The first time we discussed children was after we decided to get married (about three minutes after, actually . . . I suddenly realised, 'Oops, maybe we should have talked about this!'). I was really happy when it transpired that he was very open to the idea of having a family, and it was then that I allowed myself to start thinking about having a baby again.

Mario, who was born in Split, Croatia, and raised in Sydney since he was a baby, had also lived a full life, travelling the world as a professional tennis player. He told the *Australian*

Women's Weekly that he turned down the job of art director of a big-name design agency in New York to stay in Australia with Juanita. 'My priorities had changed and it was more important to nourish my soul than my bank balance,' he said.[1]

Eight months after Mario proposed, the couple was married on 25 April 2003. Juanita was already pregnant with Marcus. In eighteen months she had gone from being a high-flying single news anchor to being married and pregnant. No wonder she remembers well the words of the banker she met at that party in London.

During her thirties, Juanita was well aware of the debate in the media about women having babies late in life and the fact that a woman's fertility decreases with age. As a result, she was worried about her chances of getting pregnant at the age of 39.

> *I had read all the newspaper articles about this and it did concern me and it also quite depressed me. From the age of 35 women are bombarded with the message that you have to do it now or you will miss out. There was no reason for me not to believe that. I had read the articles, and basically once you hit 40 you virtually have no chance of getting pregnant.*

Then there were the negative undertones in the media about the increasing number of professional women who were leaving motherhood until their mid to late thirties.

> *There were, and still are, key messages in the media that women are delaying having children because they are selfish and they want to pursue their career and want a nice house and material goods. I think that is a complete fallacy. I know in my case, and*

*all my friends who are career women and don't have children, it
is largely because they have not had the right opportunity. Just
about every woman wants to have a child, and given the right
circumstances – finding a good man who wants to have children
with you – they will. If you find that, then a lot of women I know
would walk away from a career. This selfishness theory is quite
toxic for women but it is a reflection of the society we live in.
I think women realise they want to have a baby, but they are not
going to force themselves into poverty as a result of having a child.*

The frustration of trying to find the right man with whom
to start a family is a feeling Juanita knows only too well. She
spent eight years in two relationships from the age of 30 to 38
with men who were vague about having children and happy to
dither on the issue. Holding Marcus and knowing how costly
this procrastination could have been, she is adamant that
younger women who want children should not wait for the man
they think is Mr Right to make up his mind.

*It's hard to know what to say to young women because you want
them to have a career, but they can so easily miss out on having
a child. I think women will have children if they are with the
right partner, but when you are in your thirties with a career it
is a very scary time if you want to have kids. It is hard to meet
the right partner. A lot of men – not necessarily men I have gone
out with – have said to me that they avoid women in their
thirties especially in their mid to late thirties, because they know
these women are on a baby deadline and they don't want to be
put under pressure.*

They say if they go out with a 36-year-old woman they know that in two dates she will say, 'I want to get married and have children and not necessarily right away, but if it is not on your radar can you let me know that now?'

They find this takes a bit of spontaneity out of the relationship and I can understand the pressure they feel, but I can also understand the woman's point of view: don't waste my time as I could waste two or three years tiptoeing around the fact of wanting children.

That is what happened to me. I was in one relationship for five years and three years in another from the age of 30 to 38.

I always said to my younger women friends in their early thirties at CNN: do not waste your life on men who don't want children. Don't do it. Don't do what I did. Or you will end up at 38 once again leaving a relationship with a man who goes, 'Oh, I want to have kids eventually but not right now.' You hang around and hang around. I don't want to come across as some sort of calculating woman, but it is scary when you are in your thirties and you want to have children. Because men can have children later — they are not on a deadline.

Luckily for Juanita, Mario did not have the word 'procrastination' in his vocabulary. After he proposed a mere seven weeks after meeting her, he said he also wanted children. They proved, in a reproductive sense, a perfect match.

The fact is we decided to try for a baby, I went off the pill and I fell pregnant six weeks later. There were no problems for me. I know, though, that a lot of older first-time mothers are having problems and I am sad to hear this. But I have to wonder, too, if they are women who would have had problems earlier, but they have only come to light now because they are trying to have children in their late thirties. I don't think this is a simplistic problem.

Although Juanita had no trouble falling pregnant, felt fit and happy throughout her pregnancy and ultimately delivered a healthy baby boy, she says she was concerned and angry about the treatment she received from some members of the medical establishment when they learned her age.

Because Juanita was 39 when she fell pregnant with Marcus, who was due three days before her fortieth birthday, she was termed an 'elderly primiparae' ('primiparae' means a woman who is giving birth for the first time). It may seem strange or even offensive for women not yet forty to be termed 'elderly'. Certainly, Juanita felt that way. 'You'd think I was 110 and having an aardvark,' she commented.

When I rang the hospital the first time to arrange an appointment and they found out that (shock, horror) I was 39, they whisked me into genetic counselling. Within days I had jumped the queue and was in front of a hospital therapist telling me that I was at high risk of having a baby with a birth defect because of my age and had I considered that at my first ultrasound there was a possibility the baby may have died, and how did I think I might react to that?

I was really surprised by this attitude and a bit annoyed and I felt it was alarmist. They also strongly suggested that I have an amniocentesis and a variety of other tests.

Instead of amniocentesis, a test at 16 weeks to detect foetal abnormalities such as Down syndrome which involves taking a sample of fluid from around the developing baby, Juanita decided to have chorionic villus sampling (CVS). This is a diagnostic scan to check for genetic defects carried out at 12 weeks gestation. A small amount of the tissue that attaches the foetal sac to the uterine wall is removed through the abdomen or the vagina. The risk of miscarriage is negligible compared with the risk associated with amniocentesis, which is 1 in 200.

Juanita had the CVS at 11 weeks and an ultrasound at 12 weeks. Once again it was suggested she see a genetic counsellor. Happily, the CVS results were clear and showed Juanita was carrying a healthy foetus.

Juanita continued to read the news at the ABC until a month before the baby was due on 1 October 2003. Juanita was hoping that she would celebrate her fortieth birthday with the birth of her child, but nature had other ideas. Her birthday came and went.

Juanita had planned to have a natural water birth assisted by midwives at the Royal Hospital for Women's Birth Centre. In July 2003, when she was 30 weeks pregnant, she had quipped that her plans might go awry. Juanita was right to think that way. For starters, Marcus was almost two weeks overdue when she went into labour. Her firstborn, it seemed, was going to be late-breaking news.

He was also determined to make some headlines. After Juanita had endured sixteen hours of labour and suffered intense pain, her obstetrician decided to perform an emergency Caesarean.

Around twelve hours into labour the midwife started saying I wasn't dilated enough so she broke my waters. The contractions had started coming furiously and intensely. I had four more hours of that. She checked again and there was nothing happening so she asked if I could keep going. I said I didn't think I could for another four hours. If I was 8 or 9 centimetres dilated I would have been happy to go on, but I was only 3 or 4 centimetres. I really wanted an epidural. They took me to the delivery suite and once I had the epidural the baby went into distress. His heart rate slowed because his oxygen level dropped. By that stage we just wanted to have him born and the doctor said we have to do something now. It all happened very quickly.

Marcus was eventually born at 9.40pm on 16 October. He weighed a whopping 4.5 kilograms.

I was happy with that birth process and happy that I went through the labour. Some people said to me, 'You poor thing, you wasted sixteen hours, you should have had an elective Caesar.' But I am really glad I didn't because I wanted to experience that. It was an exciting, wonderful time for all of us.

Juanita says the full impact of motherhood is yet to hit her. Although it was only a month after Marcus's birth when we spoke, she and Mario had already experienced the confusion and anxiety of first-time parents and have had to reassess how they deal with their time and their feelings.

People told me it would be difficult and it has been difficult. I don't actually feel like a mother yet — I feel like someone has given me a baby. I feel like my normal self, but it does feel strange. I am gradually getting more comfortable with it. Then there is that sense of responsibility of being the mother. Even if my mum was there with me and Mario was there, often things would happen and they would look at me to do something about it. Marcus would have a rash and I'd say: 'Don't look at me, I don't know what to do about it!'

I really love him and I remember after the emergency Caesarean and going through that trauma and drama and just waking up the next morning and there he was in that little crib beside the bed. I remember feeling very happy and wonderful.

Juanita had made the decision before Marcus was born to return to work in January 2004. By that time, she'd had a total of five months off work, which was a combination of paid maternity leave, unpaid leave and holidays. Marcus was thirteen weeks old when she returned to work.

Juanita considers herself lucky (there's that word again) to have had time with Marcus before she returned to work. She believes strongly that working women need to have access to this kind of leave. She says it is 'inhuman and brutal' to expect women to have a baby and go back to full-time work within weeks. In Australia, all female employees, whether full-time or part-time, are entitled to twelve months unpaid maternity leave. However, according to the ABS, only about 40 per cent of female employees are entitled to paid maternity leave. Over the past two years debate has been intense over the issue of universal taxpayer-funded maternity leave, with the federal government's own Sex Discrimination Commissioner, Pru Goward, in 2002 advocating a scheme that awarded fourteen weeks paid maternity leave for all employed new mothers. This year the federal government eschewed a maternity leave scheme, opting instead for a one-off $3000 Maternity Payment for every mother on the birth of a child, after 1 July 2004, rising to $5000 by 2008.

I really feel for those women who don't have paid maternity leave and are forced to take unpaid leave. Society tends to think that having a baby is a woman's problem – you have the baby, you want to work, well, then it is your choice to work it out. But it is not just the woman's problem – it is a family problem and Australia's problem. Women are made to feel that it is their fault, but what are they to do? The country wants our taxes and it wants our productivity and it also wants us to churn out kids without giving us any support in the sense of looking after children when they are born and having more time to breastfeed them and care for them. It is just bizarre and cruel and anti-women. I hope it changes – I think it is starting to.

For Juanita, going back to work was always a matter of when, not if. She half-jokes that living in Sydney with a mortgage it is impossible for most couples to have only one partner working. As George Megalogenis notes in his book *Faultlines: Race, Work and the Politics of Changing Australia*, most women would prefer to stay home for some period of time after having a baby.[2] The problem is, they can't afford to. According to the 2001 Census, most women went back to work when their youngest child was one to two years old, and 51 per cent of all mothers were employed. Megalogenis points out that this pattern had changed in just five years – in 1996 the typical mother returned to work after her youngest child turned three.

In the 1970s a typical mother with two children spent up to a decade at home.

The nature of Juanita's profession also exerts a pressure which is just as hard to ignore as the mortgage. Television tends to have a very short memory when it comes to its employees, even those with a high profile. She went back to reading the 7pm news for the ABC in Sydney, which meant doing a full working day, starting at 2pm and finishing at 9.30pm.

It was a wrench, but Juanita says she wanted to return to work as it has been part of her life for so long and she enjoys it.

I am really lucky that I love my job and the ABC has been really supportive. I will be interested to see how I feel about not being with Marcus. I am one of those women who wants that other side of my life there again. I don't actively miss it, but it is a big part of me.

The suggestion of some kind of formal child care for Marcus was quickly tossed aside by Mario's family. Juanita remembers how her talk of having a nanny or putting Marcus into a child-care centre horrified her relatives. They didn't want a stranger looking after Marcus and so they all put up their hands to be his carer.

Since Juanita returned to work in January 2004, Marcus has been cared for by his 'baba' or grandmother, Marija. Juanita is happy knowing that Marcus is being looked after by family.

I feel extremely lucky, not just for myself, but to have this sort of practical support for my son — he is now part of this big, close community that will always look out for him.

Mario's family's views on childcare were in contrast to Juanita's. She had assumed she would put Marcus into care when she returned to work. But, as Juanita has found since marrying Mario, the Croatian community in Sydney has a traditional European attitude to family and babies. They prefer extended family to care for young children in the home rather than the use of paid childcare. Juanita also encountered different experiences of motherhood, especially among the women in Mario's family who became mothers as young women. Her mother-in-law, Marija, had Mario when she was nineteen. She is now 57.

When she had him it was still very much the tradition in that part of Croatia for women to stay in bed for forty days after they had a baby, while their female relatives and neighbours did the cooking and cleaning for them. All the mother had to do was take care of her baby. This is what Marija did – although she tells me that on day 41 her mum had her out of bed and cleaning curtains!

Mario's aunt and Marija's sister-in-law, Mirjana, was also a young mother, married by proxy in Croatia at the age of fourteen when she was still in Year 8 at school. She came to Australia when she was fifteen to join her husband, Mladen, had her first baby at sixteen and another two by the time she was twenty.

Juanita's life and her path to motherhood could not be more different. What then did Mario's family make of Juanita, who had her first child so late in life? Juanita laughs and says, 'They just treat me like the younger generation.'

Having had Marcus at 40, Juanita is one member of her generation who, in her words, managed to get 'through the door' to motherhood. She stepped off the career rollercoaster, found Mario and had a baby late in life. She's a happy woman, but can't forget those 'scary' years in her late thirties when her life choices had brought her to a point where she was successful in her career, yet a certain fulfilment eluded her.

There are all sorts of difficulties facing women who want to have a career and a family, particularly when you get into your thirties. I don't know how any woman manages to have everything, to really fully experience their relationship and have a career and have a baby. It is all so incompatible. And after you have had a baby you realise how your priorities change, that the baby comes first. It struck me the other day. I thought: 'I am going to be the most important person in his life and he is going to love me more than anyone else, not necessarily because I am me – but simply because I am his mother'. It really hit me that even when I am dead and gone and he is 80 years old he will remember me.

Alannah Hill

fashion designer

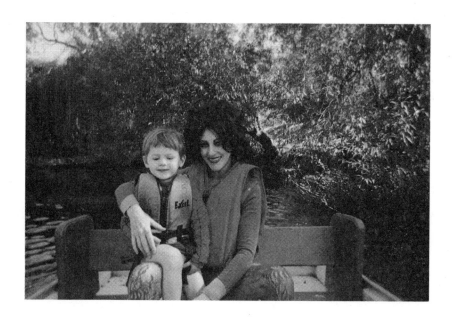

‘It's hard to hear that one is too old at 38 to have a baby because the unfortunate thing with arriving at this age is that one does not feel it. I have a lot of energy and I never lolled around in bed all day.’

ALANNAH HILL ISN'T joking when she says she doesn't like surprises. She is the reigning queen of Australian romantic fashion, her designs oozing femininity from every ruffle. However, when it comes to self-preservation, Alannah is definitely no softie. She likes to know exactly where she stands and will do whatever it takes to remain on her feet.

When she discovered in 2001 that she was pregnant at the age of 38, the first thing Alannah did was ring a specialist and arrange to have an elective Caesarean. Her next move was to find out the sex of her baby. It's tempting to suspect this was partly so she could start thinking about some frothy creations for her child-to-be's wardrobe. And it's true that once Alannah learned she was having a boy she immediately set about creating a heavenly wardrobe for her son to wear the minute he came into the world.

However, there were other reasons Alannah wanted to know exactly what she was in for when it came to first-time motherhood.

I don't care for surprises and an unplanned birth filled me with a fear I couldn't place. It all seemed a little ill-mannered and rough and I didn't want to be at the mercy of the forces of nature. I wanted to have a baby, not to endure some torturous childbirth. Horror stories of tearing just seemed ungainly and not very feminine. So a Caesarean really seemed the only sensible thing to do. I talked to my obstetrician and she told me it was the only way to go. I was thrilled with her response.

Alannah's dislike for surprises was particularly acute during her pregnancy because circumstances had made her realise that she couldn't rely on other people for help. There she was, a successful fashion designer with seven stores around Australia, having dreamed of this kind of glamorous life when she was a teenager pumping petrol at her parent's service station in Tasmania. Her signature label was a hit after a decade of dedication and hard work. And now she was pregnant. This was a time in her life when Alannah should have been celebrating and, publicly, she was the pretty picture of success. However, privately, her life was in chaos.

The disharmony stemmed from her long-time partner's unfavourable reaction to her pregnancy. Psychologist Karl Bartl, Alannah's partner for eleven years, was nine years younger than her and he did not want a child. He was busy and successful and believed he could afford to wait a few years to father a child with Alannah.

Alannah, on the other hand, was nearing her forties and knew that, biologically, it was now or never if she was to become a mother. After years of actively ignoring motherhood, at 37 she couldn't think of anything else.

I had felt so terribly sad then because I really did want a little bubba. Unfortunately, my eleven-year relationship was not ready for it; we were supposedly engaged but that was basically a sham. So . . . we had the talk. We had a lot of talks! He knew I wanted a family, we made a plan and he understood that it was important to me.

His response was something like: 'I'll do this with you but I cannot promise anything. I don't know how I will be. I think I may be distant. In fact, I will be distant. I may freak out. I may want to run. I don't want to have to support a family. If you want to do this you have to be responsible for it all.'

It was a terrible blow to hear this. His attitude towards family life tormented me for months to come. I was so bitterly disappointed and knew deep inside that I was on my own and that things would never be right with him again.

Now, any normal girl would have seen the signs. I remember thinking, 'He seems quite interested in all, well some, of this! Oh, he'll get used to it. He'll love family life!' I was in denial and blinded myself to the bad signs.

I see now that I was in a deluded state. I have since read somewhere that this is common among girls who want a baby and their current partner is the only one available. So I did it. Everybody was against it and thought me irresponsible. I didn't care. I knew it was right. Right for me. And right for Edward . . .

He would get home at six in the morning and if questioned would threaten to go out immediately again. Told me I wouldn't allow him any autonomy. He wanted to concentrate on having fun rather than working. He explained in the nicest possible way that he really didn't want to be at the birth as he would probably be seeing a band the night before and would be a little too tired. He had freaked out, but ahead of schedule. Something I had suspected and now I had to deal with.

I was having an ultrasound every two weeks to check the baby. I really couldn't fathom that a baby was growing inside me. I was always shocked and dismayed when I saw the little egg glowing on the screen and I used to laugh out loud and wonder what the hell I thought I was doing.

I tried to cover my loneliness and fear from the nurses as I knew they wondered where my partner was. I remember coming out of the doctor's one night at 8pm and there was a note on my car. It said, 'I love you more than you know. Love Karl.'

Alannah is telling this part of her late-baby story two years after Edward's birth in October 2001. Already I am getting the feeling that she is a survivor who can call on a good deal of emotional strength when she needs to. She is at work in the Melbourne office of her fashion empire and not altogether happy about her last sighting of Edward, whom she had left that morning at a local crèche.

Edward started crèche just two weeks ago. He calls this 'cool' [school]. I did the orientation and spent eight hours with him adjusting, but it is terribly hard to leave him.

He doesn't know other kids and he is unused to being around them as none of my friends have children. I guess I'm a bit old-fashioned and would love to just be at home to watch him. Everybody tells me crèche is good for him. Except my mother, who says I have ruined *him.*

When I left him bawling at the crèche for the first time I feared she might be right. I cried in the lift for minutes. I'll give it another two weeks and if I don't see him settling I will think of something else. He's only there two days a week.

And it's a good crèche. I know it will be good for his little character and well-being, but I find it unbearable seeing him so upset.

Figuring out what to do with Edward, who, up to this point, had been looked after by a nanny at home, is just one of the challenges facing single mother Alannah. Since Edward was born, she has slashed her workload dramatically to four days a week, starting at 10am and finishing at 4pm. However this routine can change as a result of Alannah's perfectionism. If she sees a display or a design she isn't happy with, she immediately moves to change it. Once, before Edward was born, she was on her way home from work at about 11.30pm and didn't like what she saw in her Alannah Hill Chapel Street store window. So she stopped and fixed it before finally heading home.

This kind of single-minded attention to detail, coupled with a determination to get what she wants, has shaped Alannah's life since she was a child. It explains why, as an older mother, she went ahead and had her child even though her partner was against it. Just as, when she finally fell into the thrall of motherhood, all she wanted to do was get pregnant.

I really was quite determined. I couldn't let anything or anybody stop me. I remember being most disappointed every month [when she menstruated] and hearing that little screaming sound in my soul telling me that it may not happen. God was going to punish me for something I did when I was small and he would repay this by not allowing me a child.

It must have taken all the determination she could muster to imagine a life outside Penguin, a timber town on Tasmania's north coast, where Alannah spent most of her childhood. Her mother, Aileen, and father, James, owned a milk bar and service station there. Alannah and her four brothers and a sister worked seven days a week, all of them pumping petrol after school and serving behind the counter. Alannah desperately needed to get away from this life. As she told *Who* magazine in August 2003, she felt 'just plain and I ran towards anything to get love. I wanted attention and to be special at something.'[1]

At fourteen, she ran away, briefly, with the circus — Ashton's Circus, to be precise. She stayed for four days, cleaning out the monkey cages and sewing sequins onto costumes. And although she went home to her parents, Alannah knew her life was elsewhere. Three years later she arrived in Melbourne, aged seventeen, with $30 in her pocket. She started work as an apprentice hairdresser and appeared as an extra in the cult movie *Dogs In Space*, which starred the late Michael Hutchence. She found part-time work as a salesperson for the Indigo boutique in Chapel Street, working her way up to being offered her own label for Indigo. In 1996, seventeen years after she left Penguin, she launched her own Alannah Hill label. If Alannah had wanted an escape route she had certainly found one in her dizzily dreamy clothes made of lace, velvet and satin.

The fashion industry can be all-consuming, and to establish herself as a designer Alannah often worked up to 70 hours a week during her thirties. There was no time to even think about having a child. Besides, she says that when she was younger she didn't want to have children because she thought parenthood was for other people. Alannah still wanted to be different.

I had always found being a mother too normal. I thought having children was for other people. People who were at peace with themselves and who deserved it. I was on the margins. Just looking in. Not really part of any group. An outsider who thought she was on the inside. I didn't really know anybody who had children in Melbourne; I had never even held a baby.

Once, a little while back, I tried to and it really did scream. The mother told me my red lipstick frightened it so I always believed I frightened children. I genuinely did not have a clue. But I quite liked that. Not having a clue didn't have to be bad, I thought!

So what changed her mind about becoming a mother? After years of saying to herself that motherhood was far too normal a pursuit for her, why did Alannah suddenly decide she wanted to be a mum?

She says originally her change of heart had nothing to do with the biological clock and the fear that she might be running out of time. She says she didn't really know much about how age can erode a woman's fertility, although she had a pretty good idea that she needed to start trying before her forties.

She says that she never had any fears that she wouldn't conceive. 'I just knew that I would get pregnant,' she says simply. Just as she knew that she needed to have a child. She also felt physically young.

It's hard to hear that one is too old at 38 to have a baby because the unfortunate thing with arriving at this age is that one does not feel it. I have a lot of energy and I never lolled around in bed all day.

I was always up and dressed and made up by 8am and I am not a party person. I had stopped going out so I was ready for that part of being a mother. I started having crazy maternal urges which were unusual for me. I would cry when I drove past South Yarra Primary School in Melbourne, cry when I saw mothers kissing their children, cry when I looked over at families in their shiny cars.

I would sit up in the loungeroom and imagine a toddler walking in and me giving him/her a little chocolate biscuit. I imagined a toddler walking around the house with me. Holding its hand and talking to it. But my life was in a safe pattern and I tried to ignore these thoughts.

I woke up one day and felt demented for six months. I really did feel a physical ache inside me and I cannot explain it. It is a mystery. I guess you could say that I felt I had everything and the relationship I was in made me curious. I started asking that gnawing question: 'Where to from here?' – a partner's nightmare!

Alannah fell pregnant after about six months of trying to

conceive. It should have been a happy time; instead she was fraught with anxiety. She was deeply troubled by Karl's opposition to fatherhood. Alannah felt increasingly alone and isolated. These feelings were compounded by her insecurity about motherhood.

She did not have a close relationship with her own mother and this had left her unsure about how she would cope as a mum. She says now she felt almost ashamed to think she could even hope to be a mother. So Alannah decided to hide her pregnancy at first, disguising it with special clothing. Designed by her, of course.

When I was pregnant, I felt dissociated from myself. I started to feel that I didn't deserve to be a mother. I was most disheartened by my partner's behaviour and really didn't know what to do.

The words 'mother' and 'mum' had always filled me with chaos and dread. It was a huge deal for me to have my own child. I started feeling very embarrassed and ashamed of being pregnant. I hid it with special clothes that I designed myself.

Looking back, I would never do that again. I would be much more at peace with it. I really don't want to blame anybody, but having a partner who I knew was freaking out and finding me gross and ugly really didn't help. To him, I was just fat. I kept asking myself, 'Who do you think you are bringing a baby into this world?'

The last three months of carrying a baby was probably the loneliest, longest and most difficult period of my life. I knew I may not have any support and quite simply, I was out of my depth and terrified. My sister was as against the baby as she was against my partner. Mum was hysterical in a paddock in Tasmania and had told me she could not help me. She was far too old and unable to travel. I was isolated and found my heart sinking and drowning and it would not stop turning over and over and giving me giddiness.

My business partner was most alarmed and kept trying to organise nannies and help, but I couldn't face any of these tasks. Sometimes I thought I could bring Edward everywhere with me. Thought it would be easy. Other times I thought a nanny could do it all. I wasn't aware of the fierce and unholy love that would come over me.

I deliberately pushed myself to work even harder. I stayed back at work longer than anybody. I wore high heels the entire time.

I had a horror of falling apart and being ordinary and would go to great lengths to pretend that being eight months pregnant meant nothing special. I worked right up until the day of the Caesarean.

These emotional difficulties were exacerbated by ill health during her pregnancy as Alannah became anaemic, making her feel weak. Then there was the fact that she would have to go to hospital. Any concerns Alannah may have had about the pregnancy and birth were compounded by her worries about losing her privacy there.

Alannah is an extremely private person. Only a few people have seen her without her make-up. Also, the designer in Alannah had a natural disinclination to wear a drab hospital robe. We are talking about a woman who doesn't own a pair of trousers and only started wearing trainers when she realised

pushing a pram was too hard in high heels. Combine this with
a mania for keeping up appearances and it's easy to see why
going into hospital was a fraught experience for Alannah.

*I went into hospital with the entire loungeroom from home. I was
afraid of hospitals and I get most unsettled in ugly surroundings. I took my special embroidered bed cover with lamps to
match. I had made Edward strange Little Lord Fauntleroy suits
with ribbons and bows. I had two suitcases full of clothes for
myself. Clearly, I was in a bit of a state, and for the first time
in a long, long time I was out of control and not knowing what
to wear.*

*I had to be at St Vincent's Private Hospital at 6.30am. They
allowed me to wear full make-up and a flower in my hair during
the operation. Karl drove me to the hospital in silence. He wore a
suit. I had bought him a 1969 gold Rolex watch the day before
as a celebration for our child's life. He had it on his wrist.*

*His face was grave and white and I stared wildly out the
window and didn't cry when we drove past South Yarra Primary
School. I think he may have held my hand. I'm not sure.*

Alannah was worried that being in hospital would threaten
her signature head-to-toe girlie glamour. She was also terrified
by the thought that in a few hours she would be holding a baby
– her baby.

*I really could not believe that they would ever hand me a baby.
When they handed Edward to me I was in some sort of la la
land shock. I looked at Karl and saw his fear. I knew then he
was going to run.*

We had a camera and the film got stuck. I became frantic as there are no photos of me until I was fourteen years old and I didn't want this to happen to Edward. The camera was whirring and not flashing and I took this to be a terrible sign.

Along with the drugs they gave me for the Caesarean I felt my first-ever anxiety attack looming over me. I kept looking at Edward in disbelief and I knew I would love him forever, although all I felt at that time was a quiet and strange bomb going off inside me.

I told the nurses I felt panic and anxiety. They gave me more drugs. I became worse and Karl went off to work. I didn't see him for a whole day after that. He didn't want to stay in the hospital with me and didn't want to see any visitors.

I do yearn for privacy and a hospital ward is the least private place of all so I was most anxious, and learning how to breast-feed and not being able to get out of bed for days was strange and alien to me.

A nurse told me harshly that she had 'no time for anxiety and you've just had a baby so get on with it'. I complained about her and never saw her again. Other nurses were more understanding.

If Alannah had hoped that having Edward would bring her and Karl together, she was to be gravely disappointed. Karl left Alannah when Edward was a newborn baby. She was devastated and immediately called her sister, Mary-Ellen, who has since become like a second mother to Edward.

My sister, Mary-Ellen, filled the gap Karl left like a perfect tiny jigsaw puzzle. We were never closer. We had lost our father only a year earlier and we were both still grieving his death.

I remember at Dad's funeral I whispered in Mary's ear that I had to create a life for his death, and I know we both looked on Edward's arrival like a little miracle.

Despite Mary-Ellen's loving help, the lack of emotional support from a partner has created a hole in Alannah's life, which she says she still finds hard to fill.

When you haven't been a mother before you learn to deal with the loss of the partner. I see other couples with kids in parks, and I do tend to let my mind wander and imagine what it would have been like with the dad around. It has always just been Edward and me, and I've learned to accept the hardships that come with being a single parent.

Your life, as you knew it, has now gone. And that is hard.

You really just cannot go out anywhere. If you do it has to be planned and organised and sometimes this is fraught with such negatives that you end up staying in for days on end.

The entire responsibility is yours and even though this is extremely difficult I have learned to see the good side. I don't have any fights in the home. No bloke telling me that Edward may be a poof if I keep letting him paint his toenails red!

Or that he is too spoilt! That he's [the partner's] not getting enough sex. That he feels left out. No fights about his food, the way he does things, the way I do things, the way we do things together. It's kind of special and lovely to have Edward to myself, really.

This may sound selfish and odd but we are as close as you like. Mary-Ellen says, 'You're all he's got,' and this sometimes makes me sad for Edward, but if one believes in fate, well, this is how it's meant to be for now I guess.

Indeed, being a single mother at 41 is not exactly what Alannah had planned for her life. However, after Edward was born her natural strength kicked in. She was determined to make it work despite what everybody had said about her decision to become a mum.

Of course, she says, she would love to find a man who loves her, but in the meantime she's happy to enjoy what she's got. And that is Edward, the centre of her life. He has even managed to usurp her long-held passion for fashion.

Before Edward was born, fashion design and making a name for herself in the industry were the priorities in Alannah's life. However, things have changed. She still designs up to 500 pieces a year, but now she makes sure there is balance in her life between work and home.

I am obsessed with him. I am in love with him. I am usually totally focused at work but when Edward comes in my world turns upside down. I do spoil him with oodles of understanding, love and compassion. People say I give him far too much attention and between my sister and I we are creating a terror, but I can't help it. Quite simply, I see him and then I give him everything.

I think it's the least a mum can do. Kids love affection and attention and I know what it feels like not to have these basic needs met. I don't want Edward to feel that isolation and coldness.

Even so, Alannah says she never considered stopping work after Edward was born, even if she wanted to be close to Edward.

I couldn't give up my work. It's really not like work any more. It has fused into something that I need and love and the Alannah Hill brand and its success mean the world to me. I really do need all that goes with it and without it I would go a little nuts!

I also have to feel financially independent – I have never had a bloke looking after me in that way. I couldn't bear to be financially dependent on somebody else. It would eat away at me.

Being established as a top designer has given Alannah some leeway when it comes to juggling work and being with Edward. For example she brings him to work with her for a few hours a couple of times a week. She says this flexibility in the workplace is one of the advantages of being an older mother. As well as the fact that she is the boss of her own label, her years of experience mean she can sketch her designs quickly and then rely on her pattern-makers to finish the job.

I was worried about how the business would perform with my interests being challenged with a newborn. I still do all the designing and attend every meeting. My team are my strength and I'm lucky they are all loyal and genuinely care. Edward is in at work a lot and I know when head office see him go for the drum and drumsticks they want to scream. I do get anxious sometimes when he is obviously disrupting their work but they are pretty good at hiding it and understanding my situation. I do get the disapproving sighs sometimes and I try to entertain him with something quieter. It would be impossible to take a little one into work if you weren't the boss. I know I'm lucky and my team work around me as best they can.

Even so, Alannah was to discover that maternity leave remains a vague concept in the fashion industry. She remembers she was at home on a month's leave after Edward was born when one of her business partners rang to ask when she was returning to work. She told him she had split from her partner, she had a new baby and she needed some time.

I asked my business partner if he could give me a couple of days. He was a little stern and asked me to bring the baby in and just be there. Work needed me and what's more, he could hear in my voice that I needed work.

Pushing a pram around on my own – without high heels! – in St Kilda, coping with a newborn and the loss of Karl . . . Well, I must have sounded a little forlorn! I would wait – sobbing in many cafés – for Mary-Ellen to finish work and then we would tend to Edward together.

I knew we were having the times of our lives even though it was so heartbreaking. I was lucky because Edward was such a good baby and I sort of wanted to go back to work but I also was torn as I knew the importance of being in the bubble with Edward. I couldn't face getting any help and David, my business partner, was worried and unsure of how I was coping.

I wasn't depressed. I was so happy with Edward but the flipside of that was that I had gained a dear little thing but lost a partner in all of it somewhere. If I called Karl he would help. He was frightened of how small Edward was but I remember him coming and cooking me a nice meal once.

The local nurse sat Karl down when he decided he was leaving and she told him the way he could help was by cooking!

I encouraged her to be most disapproving of him leaving but she was too professional.

It was terribly seriously awful but part of me understood. He had warned me and he was alarmed at how grown-up this all was. He didn't want it and he would have been grossly unhappy and it would have been wrong to stay with me. At the time I really thought I might die of disappointment. I knew he was leaving himself really. Not me. And certainly not Edward.

He asked to come back when Edward was four months old and I did take him back for a minute. It didn't work. We didn't work any more. The internal landscape we had together was gone and we couldn't find a place to be. I did get a night nanny to help me. She would arrive at 11pm three nights a week.

I would sleep and she would tend to Edward when he woke every two hours. The pressure was on as I had 250 pieces to design for the next collection plus a fashion show. I really did need to sleep, and as any new mother says, 'Sleep, sleep, I just need some sleep!'

As she divides her time fairly evenly between work and Edward, Alannah says she hasn't had the chance to become involved in a mothers group. She says she misses the camaraderie and support such a group might offer a new mother, particularly an older one seeking advice and comfort. At least Karl has shrugged off his initial antagonism towards the situation and is now keen to share Edward's care. He looks after Edward two days each week and one night. Alannah is grateful; however, you feel it is not the way she wanted it to be.

Karl is a very different person than he was. He has accepted Edward and I know would have loved to have come back to us and tried to make it work. This will make them close and for this I am pleased. It is important for Karl to see Edward, and I would never undermine their relationship.

Nor would Alannah have changed her life to have had Edward when she was younger. There may never be a right time to have a baby; however, Alannah feels that having Edward at 38 was the best time for her. Even though, in a relationship sense, her timing was terrible.

I guess in some ways it is easier being an older mum. I was bored with my life. Creating Edward's life, in turn, gave me a life. It is a very dubious pastime to have regrets and what ifs. But I would have liked a brother or sister for Edward. I guess it won't happen now but Karl has a daughter to a childhood sweetheart so I am hoping to contact her and I know she would love to meet Edward and be sisterly with him. I do know that five years ago when my career was blossoming it would have been hard to give Edward all my attention. My thirties were a crucial time and because of the effort I put in then, I can take time now, which I guess is a little wonder in itself!

Edward has given me so much pleasure. All the clichés about having a baby are true. It's hard, it's strange, it's joyous.

People always ask me how I manage on my own and I stare back at them and I wonder myself. I only get tired when Edward goes to bed and doesn't need me any more. I don't relax and I can think on five levels at once. I wonder sometimes if I am managing and I question myself all the time and am constantly feeling guilt and worry over all I do.

One could talk for ages about how they feel about their children but it's quite simple: you really do just love them and want the absolute best for them. It is profound and pure and you know you would lay down and die for them. I honestly believe it's the purest form of love, the most uncomplicated and unconditional love you will ever find. I stand back and look at Edward and I don't care how hard it is. How lonely or frightening it is raising a little life on your own.

I am having the time of my life. In having Edward I feel as though I have unlocked something deep inside of myself, and at last everything has slipped quietly into place.

Deborah Thomas

editor, the Australian Women's Weekly

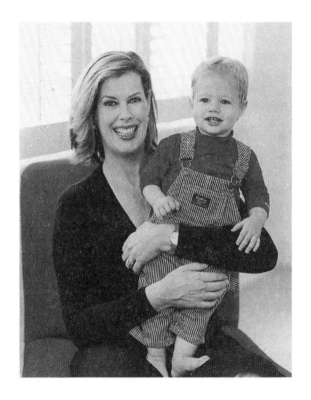

'. . . it wasn't a conscious decision either way to have children or not have children. I was just busy doing things and life ran its course.'

AS EDITOR OF the *Australian Women's Weekly*, Deborah Thomas has to be one of Australia's best-known mothers of a late baby. When she fell pregnant at the age of 45, by natural conception, the 2.7 million readers of her monthly magazine shared her joy and amazement through her regular magazine 'letter'. They followed Deborah through her pregnancy to Oscar's birth in 2002, and on to his infancy and toddlerhood.

The day I met Deborah in the Sydney offices of the *'Weekly'*, which celebrated its seventieth anniversary in September 2003, she was putting the finishing touches to a story which featured photographs of Deborah and Oscar, then 19 months, celebrating a family Christmas. Her column for this edition told readers that she, her husband, Vitek Czernuszyn, and Oscar had left their inner-city apartment for a larger home. Clearly, her role as mother is important to Deborah and while there may be no playpen in her office, she seemed determined to find other ways to soften the barriers between work and home to make the most of her relationship with the son she very nearly never had.

Since Oscar's birth, Deborah, 48, has worked hard to give her all to her job and her family, striving to maintain a five-days-a-week, 9am to 6pm work regimen. That's tough when you are the editor of the icon of Australian magazine publishing.

In an ideal world it would be nice to work four days a week, but in my job that is not really possible, so I just have to try and do my job as best I can within the hours and balance it out with my family life. Anyway, I don't think I would be very good not working. My husband says the time when I am with Oscar is so focused on him, and I enjoy it so much – I think that is because I still have time for me and my job.

Not so long ago Deborah thought time had run out for her to have a baby. It was not only her age that affected her thinking, it was also the fact that at 42 she had suffered a miscarriage. This first pregnancy had been a surprise as neither she nor Vitek had seriously considered having children. In fact Deborah was so busy with her successful career in magazines she hadn't settled into a long-term relationship until her late thirties.

It wasn't a conscious choice to have children or not. That cartoon that used to be popular which said, 'Oops, I forgot to have a baby' – that was me. Having children was just one of those things that wasn't at the front of my mind. I was so busy doing other things that I just didn't think about it. I don't know why it wasn't a priority. I just figured I'd had a very full life and somewhere along the line I had forgotten to have a baby and I had left it too late so it wasn't likely to happen. I would leave things in the hands of fate. It wasn't until I got pregnant that I realised that I really wanted to have a baby . . . and to think I nearly missed out on this amazing experience. But it wasn't a conscious decision either way to have children or not have children. I was just busy doing things and life ran its course.

Deborah was happy to let life roll along because she was getting satisfaction from her work and she enjoyed a busy social life. She had always been independent with a keen sense of the freedoms that came with having her own income. Her mother, Lola Thomas, had instilled this attitude in her daughter from childhood.

My mother worked and I never felt at any stage that we kids were not her number one priority, even though she went to work every day. What I saw with my mother was that she was a fairly independent person who had her own money and travelled a lot. I really admired her because she always knew what was going on in the world and she knew what music was happening. She would go overseas and come back with amazing things for us and one year brought back a Grateful Dead record which was pretty cool at the time.

Lola was 30 when she had Deborah in 1955. By the time Deborah was 30 she had travelled the world. She worked as a model during her early twenties after studying fine arts at

Monash University in Melbourne between 1975 and 1977. Deborah made the most of Paris in the 1970s, going to parties for fashion designers Givenchy and Kenzo, before contemplating a 'real' career. She decided she wanted to work in magazines. In May 1987 she started work as beauty and lifestyle editor at *Cleo* magazine, and went on to become deputy editor in 1990. She then moved to *Mode* magazine as editor before returning to *Cleo*, where she eventually became editor-in-chief. She moved to the *Australian Women's Weekly* as editor in September 1999.

Deborah first met Vitek more than a decade ago and after many years of dating they finally married in 1998. Not having a steady relationship until later in life was one of the reasons Deborah had not considered having children earlier.

I didn't really settle into a relationship until I was 40. Vitek and I had been dating on and off for about ten years, then I accidentally got pregnant at 42 and lost that baby. It was the crunch point as far as the relationship was concerned, whether or not we should get married. When I found out I was pregnant we decided to get married. When I lost the baby it was like, 'Are we getting married because of the baby or because we want to spend the rest of our lives together?' It was both, so we got married.

When Deborah fell pregnant at 42 she was surprised. She had thought there was little chance of falling pregnant because of her age. As a magazine editor she had overseen countless articles about women trying to have babies later in life, many of them either not succeeding or resorting to IVF or other forms of assisted reproductive technology. There were miracle births to older women, but also heart-wrenching stories of women unable to have children for a variety of reasons. The magazine had also canvassed the risks involved in late motherhood – an increased chance of miscarriage and a greater risk of genetic deformity in the foetus.

For Deborah, it seemed that even if she wanted to have a child, the biological clock was deafening in its opposition.

So her first pregnancy was a bit of a shock. Even so, she carried on working and all seemed fine. However, because she was in a high-risk category due to her age, Deborah chose to have a CVS to check for genetic abnormalities. Everything was going well, when at 22 weeks the amniotic sac started to leak and Deborah miscarried. Needless to say, it was a tough time.

I was in the hospital for two weeks trying to keep the baby and had to have an ultrasound every day to check that the baby had enough fluid. You get to know the baby very well, those little hands . . . You have this connection and when I was losing the baby all I could think about was his little feet, hands and heartbeat . . .

I asked Deborah if having a miscarriage changed her attitude towards wanting a baby. Did coming so close make her think more consciously about becoming a mother or did it make her feel it was too much of a risk?

When I first lost that baby all my hormones were going 'pregnant, pregnant, pregnant'. And you give birth to that baby and your body doesn't register that there isn't a baby in there –

even though your brain does — so at first I was running around to chemist shops saying, how do I get a fertility test, I have to get a baby back inside. Then I calmed down.

Then I came to terms with it. Everyone said how lucky I was to get pregnant late in life. Obviously it hadn't worked and I wouldn't get pregnant again. It was a one-off.

So I kind of went with the feeling that for a moment I touched it (a mother's love) and I should be happy that for a moment I knew the feeling of having a baby inside me and feeling him kick. I'd had that emotion for a minuscule moment and I was grateful for that. That is how I turned it around in my mind to live with it.

After that, Deborah says, she and Vitek didn't try for another baby.

I figured I had lost a baby at 42 and I was unlikely to ever have a baby so I resigned myself to the fact that I wouldn't. I didn't want to adopt and I would never put myself through IVF. I was quite happy to live my life without my own baby and make more of the relationships I have with children through my extended family.

Three years later, by the time she reached 45, Deborah thought that her baby-bearing days were over. Her attitude isn't surprising considering the overwhelming evidence that a woman in her mid-forties has little to no chance of falling pregnant naturally. According to the United States Centers for Disease Control, once a woman celebrates her forty-second birthday she has only a 10 per cent chance of having a baby using her own eggs – perhaps only 5 per cent if she is trying to conceive naturally.[1] The risk of miscarriage is also greater.

Deborah recalls that she didn't discover she was pregnant with Oscar until she was at the end of her first trimester. She had been feeling tired and overweight and had organised a holiday in Bali to try and get some rest and relaxation. She thought her physical symptoms were a sign of working too hard or even menopause – the possibility of being pregnant did not even cross her mind. But she became suspicious when she went out to have a coffee.

> *I couldn't think of anything worse to drink. Which was unlike me because I am a coffee addict. Then my husband suggested we have sushi and it was the same reaction. I thought, that's weird. I wonder if I could be pregnant.*
>
> *I went and got a pregnancy test – it came up positive. That was on a Sunday. I went to see my doctor on Monday and she sent me for an ultrasound – I was 12 weeks pregnant.*
>
> *My doctor said to me that this is a miracle – no one is going to believe that you did this naturally. She said this baby must really want to be here because it is against the odds.*

It didn't take a genius to work out that Deborah would be 46 by the time her baby was born. Vitek would be 49. As well as being older, he also already had a child, Sebastian, 26, from a much earlier relationship. How did he feel about becoming a father again?

> *He was as surprised as I was by the pregnancy test but it didn't take long for the idea to grow on him. He said jokingly that he*

might be too old, but I don't know how serious he was. Sure, it was something we both considered, but he got swept up in the excitement of it all.

With both Deborah and Vitek excited, if a little daunted, by the prospect of becoming parents, this time around she was determined to carry her baby to term.

I thought, 'Could I go through what I went through before with the miscarriage?' I was very conscious of that and I didn't push myself. I went home every night after work and lay down and took it easy so that there was nothing to harm the baby. I don't think the first time it had anything to do with what I did, but I was much more careful this time.

Deborah chose to have an amniocentesis at 18 weeks to check the genetic health of the child. Some form of diagnostic screening is recommended for pregnant women who are over 35, as these women are at greater risk of giving birth to a child with a chromosomal deficiency such as Down syndrome. Statistics vary, but according to the National Association for Down Syndrome in the United Kingdom, a woman aged 46 has a 1 in 20 chance of having a child with Down syndrome.

After the test, Deborah and her baby were given the all clear and she continued to work until the week before Oscar was due. It was a fuss-free pregnancy, apart from a late scare over maternal diabetes which Deborah controlled with diet.

Her relaxed attitude to childbirth may seem surprising, considering hers was such a miracle pregnancy. But it's not

Deborah's style to panic and she recalls how she had to be pushed into thinking about a labour strategy by her obstetrician.

I just thought we would decide what would happen on the day. If I needed to have an epidural that was fine. I had my bag packed and I thought we will go into the hospital and take it from there.

I think there is a lot of scaremongering about having a baby. Even the prenatal classes made you feel as if it was going to be torture and they give you the worst-case scenario. At the time I didn't feel as if I was very well informed. It was like you might throw up or you might do this or that. But it is such a different experience in the end.

Deborah worked on a Monday and Oscar arrived the following Saturday. She had thought her age might have resulted in her having a Caesarean, but Oscar was born naturally on 27 April 2002.

It's a miracle when you have a healthy baby. It is such a gift. That is what I love about my situation now. I feel like the cat who has got the cream.

I just felt immediately close to Oscar because I was so looking forward to it. When they gave him to me at the hospital he looked at me and we caught each other . . . there was this incredible feeling that this is amazing. Vitek was the same. I think he was crying.

After Oscar's birth, Deborah took four months off work. She had initially decided to take only the regular three months paid maternity leave to which she was entitled, but changed her mind. 'I just didn't feel it was the right time to come back to work.'

She then went back to work three days a week for two months and has been working full-time ever since. Having a baby has not changed Deborah's responsibilities at work. She has a demanding job, which requires constant attention to circulation figures, story quality and the performance of her staff – as well as needing to stay two steps ahead of the opposition. The women's magazine market is intensely competitive and the pressure is always on to increase readership and secure exclusive interviews with celebrities. It is hardly surprising, then, to hear that for Deborah, her toughest challenge since having Oscar has been successfully juggling work and home life.

Balancing my job and having a child – that has been the hardest part. I go to bed early. The job is demanding but I have a great team who know what they are doing. I am more organised than I used to be and I am willing to delegate more so I think I do my job better.

I am lucky because I am in a situation where I can afford to do things that not everybody can afford to do. I can afford, albeit sharing with another girl who has a baby the same age as Oscar, to have a full-time nanny at home, but it is a delicate balance. If she gets sick the whole thing comes tumbling down.

I went to a childcare centre but there were no places available. They just looked at me and said they would put me on the waiting list but I was unlikely to get anything for at least a year. I said, 'What are you supposed to do?' They said, 'You should have put him down on the list when you were pregnant.'

Vitek worked from home during Oscar's first year so he could help out and do his share of parenting, looking after Oscar by himself on Fridays. Indeed, Oscar has not only changed Deborah's life, his birth has also had many emotional ramifications for Vitek. Deborah says it has given her husband a second chance at fatherhood: 'He has a fantastic relationship with Sebastian, but they had to go through some stuff.'

The fact that Vitek is a second-time father had a positive outcome for Deborah. She says he was relaxed and comfortable around a baby. Even better, he opted for the responsibility of getting up in the middle of the night to attend to Oscar.

We have a deal. If Oscar wakes up in the night he deals with that and I do the 6.30 wake-up in the morning. He's happy to do whatever he has to at night, change a nappy or get a bottle, as long as he can sleep in at the other end.

After Oscar was born, there was no issue over whether Deborah would return to work. She says simply: 'I'm the main breadwinner so I can't give up work.' Besides, she enjoys her job – it is an integral part of her life.

For many women, returning to work after having a baby can be stressful and difficult to say the least. Is it harder or easier for older mothers?

I don't think it is an age thing. Possibly it may be easier for an older mother like me as she may be more established in her job, and I was really lucky because the company looked after me. But I have friends who are also magazine editors who are much younger and they had the same treatment when they had children. *It is not so much an age thing, it is where you are in your job and that could be any age, or whether or not the company values you.*

However, Deborah believes being older has affected the way she is mothering Oscar. She says the advantages are that she is in a mature relationship, financially well off and has plenty more patience.

I am very aware of my time with Oscar and the fact that I would rather be with him on the weekend than out partying. There is a sort of been-there-done-that feel to this kind of thing. I don't feel I would rather be anywhere else than with him. We have travelled the world, we've been to exotic locations — there is not that feeling that I would have had when I was younger when I might have felt as if I was missing out on other experiences.

Does she feel that there has been some personal sacrifice over the past two years as she has remoulded her life to become a hard-working mother of a late-in-life baby?

All I think is that it has been, and is, the most extra-ordinary change in my life. I love it on every level. It has changed my life for the better. I feel completely fulfilled. I have not made any sacrifices. It has made my life richer. Maybe I am just very lucky with the circumstances I have. Because I have a very easy baby who is strong and happy. So the word 'sacrifice' doesn't even enter my mind and it never has.

Does she feel then that she has it all – the husband, the baby and the great job? Deborah smiles before she answers.

I feel like I have it all. I have a child that I adore. I have an amazing job and a fantastic husband. It is not to say that I don't also have guilt situations when I get home from work and there is washing to do and I have a sick baby. I have all of that but I still feel as if I have it all. But it depends how you define 'all'. I am not at the Paris collections like my friends at Vogue *magazine. I have got a fantastic life that I am really happy about, but probably if you had asked me before I first got pregnant if I had it all I would have said yes.*

Articulate, successful and a first-time mother at 46 – it's tempting to make Deborah Thomas a role model for that generation of women who want to have their fun and their freedom, but also, eventually, find a partner and have a family. Indeed, Deborah has already been pigeonholed as such by the media, along with women like Cherie Blair, the barrister wife of British prime minister Tony Blair, who had her fourth child at 45.

If there is a role model thing happening, it is accidental. Because of my position on the magazine and the letter where I talk about Oscar, a lot of women have written to me and told me they have experienced the same things. It is not so much about being a role model but rather having an affinity with other women. We can talk about the same things. I love to hear about other people's lives and experiences.

For Deborah, having Oscar has brought her closer to her

readers. Motherhood has given her valuable insight into their lives and made her keenly aware of the issues that affect them, such as infertility, child care, finding the right partner and mothering.

It is funny in a way because my boss says the best thing that happened to me was having a baby. It is not so much about being a role model but having that shared experience with readers — it gives me great insight.

What it does is take me to a common point with other women who have children, whereas before I might not have understood the issues involved. I can sit down with a group of readers I don't know and start talking about Oscar or their children or grandchildren and there is an immediate connection as opposed to walking into a room as a single, childless career woman and feeling a tad disconnected. We have a common interest and you know that the things that affect you also affect a large proportion of the women reading the magazine.

This makes Deborah even more aware of the need for caution when it comes to talking about having babies later in life. She wants to be particularly careful about giving older women false hope when it comes to trying to have babies, particularly using assisted reproductive techniques such as IVF. Some glossy magazines have been criticised for their glamorisation of late motherhood and their 'miracle baby' treatment of older women who have managed to give birth using ART. Coincidentally, a late-baby story is on the cover of the *Weekly* on the day we meet in Deborah's Sydney office. The story is about swimming legend Dawn Fraser's new grandchild. The headline reads 'Dawn

Fraser's Baby Joy' and tells of the secret behind her grandson's conception. Dawn's daughter, Dawn Lorraine, 37, gave birth to her first child, Jackson Donald Fraser, after being artificially inseminated using sperm donated by a family friend. It's a classic *Weekly* yarn and the kind that brings optimism to women who are having trouble conceiving.

Deborah maintains that she is careful about giving women the wrong idea about their ability to have children later in life. When she tells her story of how she gave birth at 46, it is always delivered with a caution.

I caution women when I am asked about my situation by saying that I fall into a very small percentage of women that this has happened to. I am extremely lucky and I tell women that they need to look at all the different life stages and weigh it up for themselves and make their decision based on that information. They need to have their health records in front of them because there are conditions such as endometriosis that may affect their fertility or ability to have a baby. Women need to be across this to make their decision accordingly. I don't think there is a right or wrong time to have a child. It is up to the individual.

Yes, I had a career but I also thought if I don't have a baby, fine, I can cope with that. But on the other hand I know a lot of older women who are desperately trying to have babies on IVF and nothing is happening.

This is a complex issue that is approached too simplistically. I was lucky because I was going through life and I didn't mind either way as there was so much else going on. But there are women who really want to start a family and can't. Many of

*my friends are now in their early forties and have finally met
someone and it is too late.*

It's almost time to leave – duty calls and Deborah has to do
more work on the next edition of the *Weekly* before taking Oscar
to an appointment. We talk about her mother, whom Deborah
revealed on national television had a penchant for leather
trousers and the Grateful Dead. She remembers discussing
Marilyn French's biting social commentary from 1977, *The
Women's Room*, with her mother, who said it was essentially
about a woman's right to have a choice in life. Deborah agrees
that women must be able to make choices in their lives and be
happy with them. She says the 1970s wave of feminism and its
anthem, Helen Reddy's 'I Am Woman', was about women
saying, 'I want a whole lot of choices and I want the ability to
make that choice.'

*Which is why if someone wants kids – great. If they don't –
great. 'I Am Woman' was about defining a more complex person
who wasn't just a wife and mother. You can still be a wife and
mother but you have so much more you can do – that is what
feminism changed.*

I ask her if she thinks this plethora of choices has led some
women to enjoy busy careers, then discover in their late thirties
or early forties that they are too old to have children.

*Probably. Some . . . yes. A lot of my friends who don't have kids
say they didn't meet anyone, whether because they were too busy
working or doing this or that. I think the overriding factor is*

that they were a little like me — I just wasn't conscious of the time factor. Because look at me and my friends. As baby boomers we are eternally young. You tell us we won't climb to the top of Mt Everest at 50, and we say 'Why not?', because we're keeping fit and feeling fabulous and going to Sting and Robbie Williams concerts.

But even a baby boomer's optimism isn't enough for Deborah to consider having a second child. She says she isn't going to push her luck for another baby. She doesn't want to have IVF, and feels that having a second baby at 48 is too risky. Also, she can cope with having one child and continuing work – having two children would change everything.

Two children is a little more difficult. I did leave it late and I accept that and I am very lucky to have the little boy that I have.

Asked if this was a decision made by herself or with her husband, Deborah answers in her typical straightforward manner: 'I think nature made it for me, to be honest.'

Kerry Read

physiotherapist

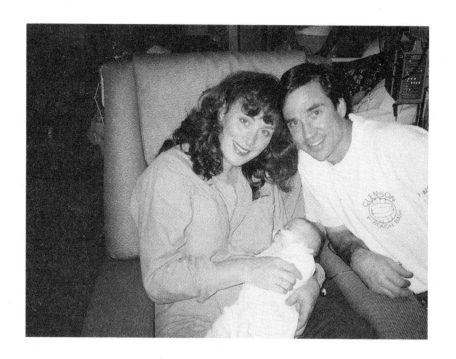

'When you think of having a child with Down syndrome you think "I could never do that", and this is what we thought. But, you know, it is just a baby and it is your child.'

IT'S LATE MORNING in Kerry Read's Brisbane home and her four-year-old daughter, Olivia, is watching a home video of herself as a baby. Forget the Wiggles or Hi-5 – judging by the squeals of delight coming from Olivia, this is definitely a viewing favourite.

Her mother is quite partial to the video as well. The footage may be the stuff of family life seen in countless other homes – Olivia as a baby being fed in her high-chair, Olivia walking, Olivia talking – but for physiotherapist Kerry and her husband, Mark Hargroder, these images represent hard-won milestones.

Olivia was born with Down syndrome, and since she was a baby, both parents, particularly Kerry, have worked hard to give her a normal and happy life. And Olivia is special for other reasons – she was born when Kerry was 43 years old and is also the first – and most probably the last – child Kerry will have with Mark, who is her second husband.

Kerry is not a high-profile women's magazine editor or a fashion designer, but her story will resonate with many Australian women, no matter their age, who have given birth to a child with Down syndrome. There may be a feeling of familiarity, too, among other women who, having separated or divorced from their first husband, went looking for another chance for a family with a new partner. This search may bring them into a world of unknowns. If the woman is in her mid-thirties or older, she may wonder if she can conceive with her new partner and then carry the child to term. If she manages to do this, how will she successfully mesh the new with the old, especially if she has children from a previous union? Finally, what if the child she has with her new partner is born with a disability or genetic defect?

Kerry, a physiotherapist, knows these questions well. They were uppermost in her mind when she met and married Mark, an engineer, in 1998. She had first married at 21, in her native United Kingdom and had two children: Emily, who was born when Kerry was 26, and Lucy, born three years later in 1986. In 1987, Kerry came to Australia with her first husband. They divorced in 1991. She spent seven years on her own as a single mum, raising her two daughters, and working to establish herself as a physiotherapist. She wasn't particularly interested in getting married again and thought that her child-bearing days were in the past.

I never had any intention of getting remarried. It was a been-there-done-that kind of thing as far as I was concerned. Then I met Mark and we had a whirlwind courtship. We got engaged three weeks after meeting. Mark had never been married and he didn't have any children and we just really wanted to have a child. It was a decision we both made. He was 37 at the time and I was 42. I just thought that he was too wonderful a person not to be a father and I also thought it would really complete our family.

Kerry's circumstances, this time, were vastly different to when she had first started a family in her mid-twenties. It had been twelve years since Kerry had given birth to Lucy. Her eldest daughter was about to finish high school. Her youngest was almost a teenager. No matter how much Kerry might have liked the idea of having another child so late in life, the reality seemed daunting.

She was also concerned about her age and the effect it might have on her ability to conceive. Also, her age put her at higher risk of having a child with a genetic defect. She was particularly concerned about having a child with the chromosomal disorder, Down syndrome.

Kerry was right to worry. Since the disorder is caused by an error in cell division, the likelihood of such an error occurring increases with maternal age. This means an older mother is more likely to give birth to a child with Down syndrome. According to figures from the National Association for Down Syndrome in the United Kingdom, a woman of 42 has a 1 in 60 chance of having a child with the syndrome. This jumps to a 1 in 20 chance by the time a woman is 46. According to Emma Bennett, president of the Down Syndrome Association of Queensland, these figures can also be applied to risk levels for older women in Australia.

Kerry says she knew she was in the high-risk category for

having a child with the syndrome, but when she and Mark first considered a family together it was not her main concern.

I was not even sure if I was still able to conceive. Actually, I thought conceiving would be a problem so it was a case of thinking that we would actually be lucky enough to get pregnant in the first place.

The possibility of having a miscarriage also worried me; however Down syndrome was also a big feature on my mind. It was something we discussed and I knew that Mark felt very strongly that we would try for a baby and then take whatever baby we got. We did not want to have a lot of testing.

Kerry says she looked for a book or some kind of information that would be pertinent to her as an older mother. She could only find American writer Sheila Kitzinger's book, *Birth Over 35*. But she wanted to know more. In particular Kerry wanted to know of other women like her who'd had, for whatever reason, a child later in life.

I guess you could say I was looking for reassurance. I wanted to see that someone had done it and it was okay, and I was concerned about Down syndrome. I suppose it would have been nice to have read about someone who'd had a Down syndrome child and that it was all okay. I did lots of homework myself. I went on this big fitness regime. I took vitamin supplements and I was super healthy.

To her surprise and joy, Kerry fell pregnant quickly. That hurdle had been cleared. However the big one was staring her in the face – this was the issue of testing. Should she have a non-invasive, low-risk screening test like a blood test or a scan or a diagnostic test such as amniocentesis which involves taking fluid directly from the placenta and is an accurate, though riskier, predictor of an abnormality in the foetus? Kerry decided that she did not want the invasive tests, opting for a scan, partly because of the risk of miscarriage that can result from an amniocentesis or CVS. And she had other reasons.

I decided to have a scan at about 20 weeks because I wanted to make sure there were no problems with the placenta which would have seriously affected the outcome of the pregnancy. Also, I didn't want to spend my pregnancy relating to a syndrome. I really wanted to enjoy my pregnancy as we had always decided we only wanted one child together.

At this point, Olivia, her hair in plaits, presents herself in front of us. Apparently the video of her baby days has finally lost its allure. A curious four-year-old, with a remarkable memory for names, she asks me, 'Where do you hurt?' 'She thinks you are a patient,' says Kerry, who has moved her physiotherapy practice into her home since Olivia's birth. She then turns her attention to her mother. 'I love you,' she says. 'I love you too,' Kerry replies. She holds Olivia in her lap while she continues her story, speaking softly but clearly.

I had the scan and it showed there were no soft signs of Down syndrome such as the extra skin-fold at the neck, but it showed she had a heart condition which can be an indicator of Down syndrome. But when I was first scanned it appeared to be a different kind of heart condition, called Ebstein syndrome, which can have a poor outcome but has no connection to any kind of genetic disorder. I found myself torn between wishing it was that rather than a hole in the heart, because if it was a hole in the heart then it was almost certainly Down syndrome. I was feeling guilty, wishing the baby had the worst heart condition it could have. But at that point I think I knew that I had a baby with Down syndrome.

Kerry says the condition was soon identified as a hole in the heart, which can afflict more than 50 per cent of children with Down syndrome. After the scan, which was attended by her daughter Lucy, then 13, and her husband, Mark, Kerry was shaken. But she did not want any more tests, especially not an amniocentesis, even though this would have indicated immediately if she was carrying a child with Down syndrome.

Kerry says her obstetrician was supportive of this decision, but there was pressure from another quarter. The radiologist who carried out the tests wanted Kerry to have an immediate amniocentesis. In retrospect, Kerry says being older and wiser as well as strong in her relationship with Mark meant they could stand by their decision not to do so.

We said no and he shouted at me: 'Don't you know the baby will probably only live for a few days – you wouldn't want that, would you?'

It was horrible. I was so worried about Lucy who came out of the room sobbing. Fortunately Mark and I had discussed this and we knew what we wanted. I think if you were wavering a bit there was no way you would have refused him. He was phys-

ically intimidating and shouting. He kept saying there was still time – meaning time to terminate. There would have been no hope for a naive 21-year-old. It would have simply been assumed you would have the amniocentesis.

The day of the scan, Kerry says she was 'a wreck'. To her surprise, Mark, after they were given the results, said he was going to his regular choir practice and wouldn't be home until late.

I could have talked for a week, but I don't think it had hit him. I don't know whether it was because he wasn't used to having family responsibilities or because he is a guy and he thought, 'Well, that's that and the baby won't be born for another 20 weeks so why worry.' I don't know what it was about because he is such a wonderful dad to Olivia. I think he assumed that Olivia would be a lot worse than she is. His picture of someone with Down syndrome, like me, was a lot worse. It wasn't someone like Olivia, who has exceeded way beyond our expectations.

Kerry emotionally and mentally avoided the issue of Down syndrome, even though in her heart she felt sure that she was carrying a baby with the disorder. She remembers that she would not look at children or adults with Down syndrome if she encountered them in the street. If she was in a train and there was someone with Down syndrome there, she would change carriages.

In the end, giving birth to Olivia was like a circuit-breaker for her emotions. Having her baby in her arms meant she could no longer ignore the reality of Down syndrome. Olivia was there in flesh and blood. Besides, by then it was a case of her parents simply being relieved she was alive after almost losing her when she was born.

Olivia was born on 28 August 1999 after a trouble-free pregnancy and labour. After having two babies, Kerry knew what to expect in childbirth. She remembers cleaning the house the night before she gave birth, having told Mark to go to bed because her contractions had stopped. They hadn't. She gave birth at 6am after a drug-free labour, having used breathing techniques she had learned at classes years before in the United Kingdom to help her manage the pain.

The midwife kept trying to talk to me which is hopeless because you can't talk when you are doing the exercises.

Clearly, this is one determined woman. After Olivia's birth, Kerry was going to need all of this determination. The baby was not long in her arms when she started turning blue as a result of her heart condition. She was taken away for treatment and tests. Any concerns Kerry had about Down syndrome were shoved aside.

We didn't think she was going to live which was good really because we didn't worry about Down syndrome. We just wanted desperately for her to stay alive.

But Kerry had seen her baby long enough to know that her previous fears about Down syndrome were correct. She had looked down at Olivia's feet and noticed a large gap between her big toes and her second toes — a telltale sign of Down syndrome.

*The paediatrician came and asked me if I had any concerns
about Olivia and I said yes, I thought she had Down syndrome.
He said he was very suspicious.*

Tests done soon after Olivia's birth confirmed that she had
the most common form of Down syndrome, trisomy 21. 'Actually
to find out was a relief,' Kerry says. 'I didn't have to run and
hide any more. There it was in front of me.'

Kerry felt relief, but she also felt terribly guilty. She asked
herself why this had happened to her and if she had been wrong
in wanting to have another child so late in life, knowing the
risks.

*I was guilty, guilty, guilty because I was old; what did I think
I was doing? I had already had my chance to have children,
what right did I have to think I could do it again and cheat
nature? Every guilty thought you could imagine, I had.*

*I look at the pictures now of me and Olivia when she was
born and I look so happy, but I don't know if I was. A lot of
women go through a grieving process when the baby is born and
men can find it very difficult to come to terms with the fact that
their child has Down syndrome. I was very fortunate with
Mark, and besides, Olivia is the only baby he has ever had. To
him she is perfect and she is normal.*

*But for me those first few weeks were hard. You do grieve.
I found it easier, though, to grieve with a baby there than
I would have done if I had gone through the grieving process
during my pregnancy. I don't think it would have been very good
for the baby. Instead, I'd just put my head in the sand and
pretended it wasn't happening.*

After Olivia was born, however, Kerry's major concern was to keep her alive. She needed heart surgery, but she also needed to be a decent weight before the operation could be carried out. She had to be tube-fed because of all the equipment needed to keep her alive, but for the first two days she could not tolerate the tube in her mouth. On the third day she was able to take the tube to be fed.

I think she just decided to stick around. So she went from being covered in leads to coming home with us. She turned the corner quickly and within eight weeks she'd had surgery.

Her hole in the heart corrected — Olivia will proudly show you the 5 centimetre scar on her chest — there were other challenges to face. Kerry was determined to breastfeed Olivia — a difficult task with many Down syndrome babies who lack the fine motor skills to suck milk from the mother's breast. As a physiotherapist who specialises in the mouth, Kerry knew that breastfeeding was best for optimum oral development and speech. It meant an extra commitment from Kerry who decided to stop work after Olivia was born to focus on her baby, at least for the short term. After she was born Olivia had to be tube fed every three hours, night and day, because she needed to gain weight. The tube feeding was supplementing breastfeeds in the two months before she had heart surgery.

If she didn't wake up we had to wake her up. It was hard work because I had to try and breastfeed her, then express and tube-feed her and then clean out all the tubes. By the time we did that it was just about time to start all over again.

Babies with Down syndrome have special needs because of their condition, which can affect every cell in the body, including the skin, bone marrow, blood and muscle tissue. It also produces more than fifty physical characteristics such as the bull neck, slanting eyes and small, low-set ears. Down syndrome babies can be prone to colds and bronchial complaints, ear infections and eyesight and hearing problems. They have low muscle tone, or a lack of tension and strength in the muscles, and are sometimes referred to as 'floppy' babies. Low muscle tone can affect fine motor skills like chewing and talking and gross motor skills like walking, running and jumping. Phsyiotherapy is used extensively when the children are young to encourage muscle-strengthening.

Learning how to help Olivia and satisfy her special needs is a never-ending journey for Kerry and Mark. So far it has required a lot of determination and love. Kerry initially struck out on her own, trying to find people to help her. She then sought advice from the Down Syndrome Association of Queensland (there is a similar association in most states), which had sent a representative to talk to her in hospital soon after Olivia was born. The association has helped Kerry source advice, through the government agency Disability Services, on how to feed a baby with low muscle tone, what to do to improve low muscle tone and how to cope with other aspects of the syndrome. In an effort to give back something of the commitment and support she has had from the association, Kerry often gives talks about having a child with Down syndrome, telling her side of the story.

To help improve her low muscle tone Olivia does gymnastics and swimming – during our interview she changes into her swimming gear and insists that both Kerry and I join her in the small pool in the backyard. Kerry, too, has worked hard on Olivia, using specially devised games to help correct problems. There is a tendency in Down syndrome children for the tongue to protrude. Kerry shows how she has worked with Olivia to correct this. 'What do we say when we put our tongue out?' she asks Olivia. 'Tommy tongue! Put it back in.' Olivia plays the game, giving a big grin at the end of it.

When Olivia was younger she suffered from pulmonary hypertension which is high blood pressure in the arteries that supply the lungs. This can cause dizziness, tiredness and a shortness of breath. Olivia had this condition from birth and it did not correct itself after her heart surgery. Kerry says there is no explanation for her daughter's condition and it is not common in children with Down syndrome, however it is more prevalent than in the general population. This was a major concern until Kerry changed her daughter's diet. Olivia now exists happily on gluten-free and dairy-free foods which Kerry says have made her daugher markedly healthier.

With Olivia at kindergarten a few days a week, Kerry has been able to return to work – and finds herself in demand. Having Olivia has made her reassess some elements of her practice, and she now specialises in teaching women how to feed babies with low muscle tone.

Kerry is confident and at ease with her child and you have to wonder if having experience as a mother gave her a softer landing when she found out Olivia had Down syndrome. She agrees this helped with the initial shock. She isn't so sure that being older has meant she's coped better with the realities of having a child with Down syndrome. Yes, she knew about the disruption a new baby could cause to the family, the sleepless nights and the endless worry. However, she did not know how having a child with Down syndrome would rearrange what she already knew about parenting. The surprise was that despite the extra effort, being older helped her feel more relaxed and patient with life.

> *I think being older you realise that life goes by in such a flash that you take more time and relish the moment more. You enjoy their childhood and are not in a rush to get to the next stage. Children like Olivia can take longer anyway so that makes for a much more laid-back approach.*

Watching her with Olivia, who is about to set off for kindergarten, I am surprised to hear that, in those early days, Kerry had certain defence mechanisms to help her cope. She remembers how she used to ignore any literature about adults or older children with Down syndrome. Anything about babies with the syndrome was okay. This was about all she could cope with at the time, and today she still says that it is best not to look too far into the distance.

> *When you think of having a child with Down syndrome you think 'I could never do that', and this is what we thought. But, you know, it is just a baby and it is your child.*
> *You don't try and cope with it straightaway. It is a day-to-day thing; it is like adjusting to having a new baby anyway, which can be just as challenging.*

Kerry says her family lives a regular life and there is little they cannot do because Olivia has Down syndrome. For

Christmas 2003 they went to America to visit Mark's family. The whole family, in particular her two older daughters, has benefited from having Olivia in their lives. Kerry says that Emily and Lucy are fiercely protective of Olivia and very proud of her. There has never been any resentment or jealousy, and Olivia considers herself lucky as she gets to see all their 'big' friends, especially the boys. Seeing the way her daughters interact with Olivia and how it has improved their under-standing of people with disabilities has also helped assuage some of the guilt she felt as an older mother when Olivia was first born.

> *I find there are benefits in my life for having had Olivia. I have become a better person. I think we all have. You have such a wider appreciation of people. I think the secret with Down syndrome or any other syndrome is how you cope. I only look as far into the future as I can manage. She is now four and a half and I am looking to send her to a regular primary school because she manages perfectly well at her kindergarten. People say to me, what about secondary school? I just don't know.*
>
> *What I can say is that having this child has opened my eyes to other things. You think, 'Why worry?' They are just a person and it doesn't really matter.*

In a follow-up interview Kerry says she doesn't want her story to sound too negative. Yes, it was tough in the early days when Olivia was born, but all new parents, no matter their age, can find a baby hard going. The tube-feeding, the worries about Olivia's health – they are all over now, leaving Kerry and Mark to enjoy their child.

I want to stress to people that I have never, for a moment, regretted the decision to have Olivia. In the early stages of her life I wished that she didn't have all her health problems, but I could never honestly say that I wished she didn't have Down syndrome because then she wouldn't be the Olivia we adore. I simply wouldn't change a hair on her head.

Lisa Forrest

former Olympic swimmer, author

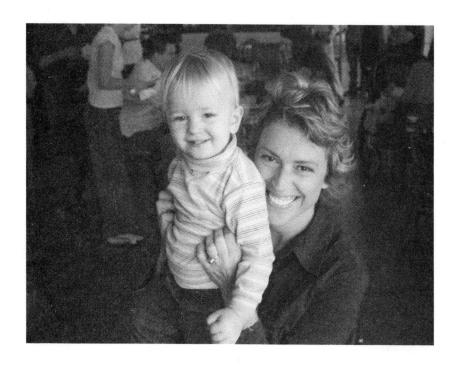

'I think there is a major conservative backlash going on out there and women are an easy target. It starts with negativity about women delaying motherhood.'

LISA FORREST HAS always been the kind of person who prefers swimming upstream. As a teenager she pushed herself to her physical limits to make the Olympic Games in Moscow in 1980 where she represented Australia in the 200 metres backstroke final. Already a Commonwealth Games silver medallist, she was just sixteen when she stood on the Olympic starting blocks.

Then, four years later, she abruptly changed lanes to work as a television reporter and commentator for the Seven Network. Six years on she decided to swim against the tide once more, interrupting a comfortable career in television to study acting. This was followed by yet another career zigzag, with Lisa deciding to pursue her dream to become a writer.

Last year, Lisa's life changed dramatically once more when she became a first-time mother at 38.

It's been twenty years since she stopped competitive swimming, yet Lisa still has the long, lithe body of an athlete. We're having a late morning cup of peppermint tea – make that trying to have a cuppa. Between sips, Lisa is constantly moving in tandem with her latest life challenge, her infant son, Dexter, who is crawling around the loungeroom of the temporary Sydney residence she shares with her husband, Jesse Todd, an IT consultant.

Dexter was born on 19 February 2003. Perhaps in early acknowledgment of his mother's creative pursuits, he made a dramatic entry into the world. At the last minute, after a long but trouble-free labour, Dexter, weighing a robust 4.5 kilograms, became wedged behind Lisa's pelvic bone. He was freed by a midwife and obstetrician using a combination of forceps and manipulation.

Nine months later, there are no barriers to Dexter's discoveries. He seems determined to walk and at the same time reach out for every object in the room. He makes a move for his mother's steaming peppermint tea followed by a lightning quick grab for a nearby lamp. Lisa's eyes never leave him, and it is easy to see why, at one point after Dexter's birth, she had to temporarily abandon the writing of her first adult novel. Actually, she recalls that the book slid to second place even before Dexter was born, when she was pregnant and not feeling the least inclined to write. After he was born, it became a challenge to focus on the solitary task of writing with a baby in the house.

By the time of our interview, Lisa had returned to work on her media projects. A few days earlier, she had been on a panel for the Foxtel network's *Mars Venus*, to talk about women and careers. She had also recently finished her monthly taping of a series of interviews for Qantas Airways' award-winning inflight entertainment channel, On Q.

It is not the typical nine-to-five, five-days-a-week work schedule, yet it is a busy life. In the past few months it had been made even more hectic by the fact that Lisa, Jesse and Dexter had been living in a variety of friends' houses while their own home, a former corner shop in inner-city Sydney, was being renovated.

Lisa doesn't seem too fazed by the somewhat erratic nature of her life; besides this is a woman who has always had – and needed – variety and challenge.

Come to think of it, motherhood sounds as if it has been the perfect salve for Lisa, whose yearning for satisfaction in life and work has led her down a plethora of career paths. Ironically, it was this constant search for satisfaction that led her to delay having a child. She was so hellbent on trying to prove to the world that she could be more than a swimmer that she dedicated herself to her profession of choice, be it reporting, acting or writing.

She readily admits her search was intensified by a need to overcome her personal dissatisfaction that followed her controversial backstroke final at the Moscow Olympics. In the split second before the starting gun cracked, Lisa, a gold-medal favourite, lost her footing on the wall. This caused her to lose the race but it meant the start of another challenge – to find contentment.

As reluctant as I am to admit it, I am highly competitive. I won't compete against others, but I compete against myself constantly. I just don't see the point of doing something, like writing a new book, unless it's different or better to what has come before.

There is even a rule in our house that I can't comment on the meal I've cooked until we've finished eating, because Jess wants to enjoy it before I tell him what I did wrong. So contentment has been rare and fleeting.

But, with pregnancy, I was swamped by contentment and even though I had guilty moments, I couldn't believe the peace and freedom it brought.

And then to put into some context that I was an Olympian at sixteen, I've always passed it off as something anyone could do if they trained hard enough. I have never accepted that I had any special talent or physical gift. But when I got pregnant I would say to Jesse how funny it was that after all those years of imposing a training regime on my body, with pregnancy it was as if it said, 'Thanks very much, get out of the way, I know what I'm doing.'

All I had to do was sit back and watch. And enjoy it because I was so well. I felt like I could run marathons. I'd go for my usual walk in the morning and often I'd swim in the afternoon as well. After an hour in the pool I had to stop myself because I'd think, 'I'm pregnant, I'm sure I shouldn't be doing this.' At a certain point I had to concede that maybe, physically, I'd been given something that not many people had.

Since she had Dexter, Lisa can count on her fingers the number of times she's been in the swimming pool. In fact, Dexter has been in the pool more than his mum, attending swimming lessons. Apparently he has taken to swimming like the proverbial duck to water. No, Lisa says, she is not encouraging him to be a swimmer, but the lessons are a great way to create a tired child and therefore encourage sleep.

For me, gliding through water is one of the most delicious sensations I know. That's all I want for him from the swimming lessons.

Lisa reveals that late motherhood has brought monumental changes to her life which have made her more sensitive to the world around her.

You are suddenly completely raw to the world. I feel as if I am just more sensitive as a person because I have this little person I am protective of. I have to rethink the way I do everything, even the most basic things. I really enjoy it but I also feel sometimes that I can't control my emotions in the way I used to be able to.

I remember thinking what an autonomous little person he is, even when he was just born. The thing that I'm shocked by is that I've never felt like I own him. He's not mine, he's just in my safekeeping until he is an adult and my job is to give him all the tools he'll need when he gets there. This was terrifying at first because I thought: 'Do I have the internal fortitude to do this? Do I have the skills?' I feel as if I am balancing all the time. I don't want to smother him with love but it is hard to resist.

And as hard as it can be sometimes, the bad times are never as awful as the good times are exquisite.

Dexter is obviously a much-loved late-in-life baby whose arrival has made Lisa think deeply about the way she lives her life and the future she wants for her son. And yet she could easily have missed out on becoming a mother as for many years she simply wasn't interested in having children.

In July 2003 she told the *Australian Women's Weekly* that, 'It took me a long time to want to be a mother. Now there are times when I think I nearly missed this and I am so glad I didn't.'[1]

So what were her reasons for delaying motherhood until her very late thirties? Just as is the case with many other women of her generation, there is no simple answer.

For many years, Lisa was busy with her different and demanding careers and in this aspect of her life, at least, she was happy, like most women are, to go with the flow. Swimming consumed her teenage years and after competing in the Olympic and Commonwealth Games she swam her last major competitive race in 1983. By then she had collected a silver medal in the 200 metres backstroke at the 1978 Commonwealth Games in Edmonton, and gold medals in the 100 metres and 200 metres backstroke at the Commonwealth Games in Brisbane in 1982. At the Moscow Olympics in 1980, where she lost her footing in the backstroke final, she had been the captain of the swimming team.

But four years later she had left behind the world of competitive swimming to work as a sports reporter for Channel 7 News and *Sportsworld*. These days many sportspeople move on to work in television as commentators or reporters, but then it was an unusual thing to do, especially as Lisa wanted to report on all subjects, not just sport. She switched to the ABC in 1986 as a presenter and reporter and also worked as a commentator at the 1986 Commonwealth

Games in Edinburgh. From 1987 to 1989 she worked for the *Midday Show* with Ray Martin as a general reporter covering stories in Australia and overseas. She continued to work in television, hosting ABC-TV's health series *Everybody* in 1992 and commentating for Channel 7 at the 1992 Olympic Games in Barcelona. In 1993 she moved to New York to study acting, then worked as a radio host back in Australia for a year and in 1996 moved to Brisbane to play the part of Marina in the Network Ten medical drama, *Medivac*.

Around about this time she decided to pursue a long-held desire to write. The opportunity to do so commercially arose two years later when she received her first book contract from Hodder Headline to write young adult fiction.

Her first book, *Making the Most of It*, a teenage novel about a young swimmer who makes it to the Olympics but struggles with the demands on her, ultimately slipping at the starting blocks, was released in 2000. She completed her second young adult novel, *djmAx*, in 2002.

Her work commitments kept her busy, and besides, Lisa had not met a man with whom she wanted to have children. She had also learned a lesson in her early twenties when her boyfriend at the time had a toddler from another relationship.

He had a little girl who was about two and you realise that you don't have any time to yourself when you are with them – you can't even go to the toilet by yourself. The other thing that was really obvious was that, with a child, it is the woman's life that changes dramatically. I think men can decide really the degree to which their life changes, but a woman's life is turned upside down.

So this experience was really instructive in the sense that I thought I would do the things that I really wanted to do before I had kids. I think this works because you do have more of a sense of self by the time you become a mum.

Having said that, I had not met the right person (with whom to have children) so there was no choice, essentially. I knew I wanted children one day but I didn't want to do it alone.

Lisa finally met the right person in Jesse, whom she married five years ago. They wanted to have children but the time never seemed to be right. Jesse was still in his mid-twenties – he was 30 when Dexter was born.

I was a bit worried about Jesse that he wouldn't be as clucky as me. But it was all in my mind and had nothing to do with him. Ever the realist, he knew that marrying a 35-year-old woman meant we'd have kids sooner rather than later. His age didn't have much to do with my late motherhood as just falling in love with him. For me, meeting the right person brought it all on.

Even so, there were a few pragmatic issues prompting them to wait for the so-called 'right' time to try to have a child.

We were having a few hassles in that Jesse was out of work and we had bought a house. He had lost his job because he rode that e-commerce wave and was dumped pretty badly by the whole thing. But then my girlfriend was diagnosed with breast cancer, and was ravaged by it really quickly. At that same time my brother's best friend died of an aneurism at 36. I just thought, 'What are you waiting for?'

Also, I don't think you can say there is a right time to have a child, but it took a long time for me to get clucky. When I did get clucky, it hit me like a freight train.

I was auditioning for a job at Channel 7 and it was a really long audition process so we just put off trying to get pregnant. It was a big job and we thought it would be worth it. I got the job but then it was cancelled because of the terrorist attacks on September 11. At that point we decided to just go for it.

Lisa says she had heard all the statistics about how a woman's fertility falls as she ages, a drop that accelerates as a woman enters her late thirties to early forties, when the chances of becoming pregnant are estimated to be only 5 per cent each cycle as opposed to 25 per cent at a woman's fertile peak in her early twenties.

I knew all this but I believe in personal responsibility. If you are going to wait until you are older to have a baby then you know you are taking a risk. You can't assume that it will all work properly.

Lisa had never been on the contraceptive pill and was fit and healthy. However she was concerned that she had not gone through puberty until she was nineteen and she thought this could have some effect on her fecundity. Also, her mother, Caretta, had taken four years to conceive her first child. But after Lisa was born her mother fell pregnant again quickly with Lisa's brother, Greg.

I think there are so many mysteries to pregnancy – it is not just about sperm fertilising an egg. It is about how you are at the time and where your head is at. There are so many things that play a role in what happens.

As it happened, Lisa fell pregnant quickly. She was surprised, because she was aware of the media reports at the time about the increasing trend to late motherhood and the associated problems of infertility.

During my pregnancy there was a lot of stuff in the media that made me really angry: stories about the need to teach girls at school about how their fertility drops off – as if you don't know that for a start. I think there is a major conservative backlash going on out there and women are an easy target. It starts with negativity about women delaying motherhood. If you believe everything you read in the media you would think that nobody gets pregnant over 35. But that is not right.

Some women do have trouble getting pregnant – but the majority don't. I think because you don't want to hurt anyone who is going through that trauma [of not being able to get pregnant] there are a whole lot of women who are whispering, 'Did you have any trouble? No? Neither did I.' I think that is one of the great secrets – there are a lot of older women who didn't have any trouble getting pregnant.

There is also a kind of media terrorism about women having babies later in life. Even the other day there was another story in the newspaper about the drop-off in fertility in Australian women and the statistics sounded really scary. But it is just scaremongering. You have to keep reminding yourself that the media loves bad news. That is what sells.

The confusion and fear that may exist among young women over the dilemma of when to have a baby have made Lisa confident that older women who experience a healthy pregnancy, either naturally or using reproductive technology, should speak out.

We need to be upfront about it because it is all about taking responsibility for yourself and the choices you have made in life. It is particularly important at this point because there is a general conservatism again in society, whereas in the 1970s there was more of a feeling that you could do everything. Now it is as if feminism is to blame, not just for women thinking that they could be a supermum, but for all of society's ills.

I was master of ceremonies at the 2003 Telstra Businesswoman of the Year and the New South Wales winner was the head of TAFE, Marie Persson, and the first thing that she said was choose your employer well — because she felt she could do both, she could have a family and she has a great career because she had a good employer. I think it is all about putting the power back in your hands.

Lisa is the main carer of Dexter and she plans to continue working on her writing and other projects. She admits that she is worried about the juggle she faces between Dexter, her book, other work commitments and maintaining her relationship with her husband. She says she worries about this balancing act all the time.

I was brought up by a mum who didn't have a career. When we went to school she worked between 9am and 3pm. She was always around for us. So I don't have an example of a mother who was out to work having her own life in that way. There are times when I think I should be giving Dex that sort of a life — not one where you have a mother who is mad for her career. Right now I don't need to put him into day care and I don't want to do that. At the moment I am just taking it as it comes. I do worry about work and how I will manage it, but I think it is important that he gets off to a good start. I will just run with it and see how it goes.

This 'wait and see' attitude has helped Lisa in the past to move between different kinds of work, and when she first fell pregnant she maintained this approach.

I do remember my closer friends calling and offering advice, plus the natural birth brigade who stirred me up about having an amniocentesis, for instance. They didn't want me to have one and I can remember saying to my doctor that I wasn't going to have one because it was a bit invasive.

She just looked at me as though I was mad and I thought, well, I had better reassess this and then actually started listening to what people were saying to me. There was often a sentence attached to one end of the advice: 'And anyway you wouldn't do anything if you found out that there was something wrong with the child.' Well, if I did find out I was having a child with Down syndrome or with one of the other chromosomal abnormalities they test for I would do something about it. Having said all that, going through the amniocentesis was one of the most amazing experiences of my life. I was so tense that I had a headache at the end of it all because of the build-up, but I was amazed by how precise it was. You could see everything, where the needle was, how the baby was coping. I found the process extraordinary.

Lisa says that during her pregnancy she was 'on cloud nine'. She felt content and happy, overwhelmed by a feeling that she had been fortunate to have 'this incredible life'.

I felt that I have been lucky to do the things I wanted to do and I had the baby and he came along at the right time. It just all happened at the right time.

However, while pregnancy was a breeze, childbirth proved to be a little more challenging. Lisa says she had not planned her labour – she just wanted it to unfold naturally, and whatever had to be done, then she was prepared to do it. She says she went to see her obstetrician on the morning of 18 February. She learned her cervix was 1 centimetre dilated and by the afternoon she was feeling some discomfort. Even so she went out to dinner with Jesse but didn't eat much because by then her contractions were starting to come in waves.

By the time we sat down at the restaurant I had to concentrate because of the contractions. Jesse said we should time them and by his calculations I was having a contraction every two and a half minutes, one for 45 seconds and one for 25 seconds alternatively.
We finally got to the hospital at 11.20pm. When I got there I grabbed the table because of this contraction and the midwife said I wouldn't be going home that night. It just went very fast after that. Around 1am I was fully dilated but the pain was

intense and I thought that to do this on my own I would have to leave Jesse and go right into myself. I wasn't interested in doing that. So I had the epidural.

Lisa remembers how she had been pushing for an hour when everyone realised there was something wrong.

He (Dexter) had come down the birth canal sideways and he was caught on the pelvic bone. I had an hour at the end of my labour that was really tough.

After four failed attempts to free Dexter using the vacuum extractor, forceps were necessary and Dexter was finally born at 6.02am. There were a few anxious moments for mum and dad; however Dexter was already taking the world in his stride – his heart did not miss a beat during the delivery. The same could not be said for Lisa and Jesse!

Lisa admits that there have been moments when she's felt thwarted by being a new mum, particularly when the writing of her first adult novel had to be shelved after Dexter's birth. This was a part of her creative self that the maturer Lisa finally felt ready to explore. It was frustrating to have this important journey stymied, at least temporarily, first by pregnancy and then by the demands of a new baby.

The thing I found most difficult after Dexter was born was that I had hardly written anything of my book. I just found it really difficult writing after he was born because I was so completely wanting to be with him. Even when I was pregnant I found it hard to concentrate on my writing. I was on cloud nine.

It has taken me quite a while to get my head around the idea of writing again since Dexter was born, but I listened to Nikki Gemmell [Australian author of The Bride Stripped Bare*] talk one day and she said she was able to find writing restorative. In the beginning, when Dexter was first born, I couldn't face it, but now I do a little bit every day and it is fine.*

It is like putting something back into my life. But it did take a little while to find that thought. It has taken a shift in the way I am telling the story so the book is going forward which is really nice, because for six months nothing happened.

The biggest change for me, though, since Dexter was born is that I went from a person who, whenever things went a bit awry, could exercise her world back into equilibrium. Lack of time, plus recovering from birth, plus breastfeeding meant that to exercise in the way I had before was exhausting me. Then, at about five months, I started meditating.

It was as if everywhere I turned there were stories about its benefits. So I tried it and became a complete convert. If you'd told me sitting still and just breathing for twenty minutes would have given me so much energy [before I had Dexter] I would have laughed and said, maybe for someone else. Even when I did yoga I did ashtanga! But one night, not long into practising it, Jesse was working late so I put Dex to bed at 7pm, meditated, then went to work on my book. Jesse got home at around 10pm and after we were talking for a while he asked when I'd had my last coffee. I said at nine this morning but I meditated tonight and he said, well your energy is amazing. Physiologically, I don't know what it does but it works for me. That's probably the most significant change.

Now that Dexter is becoming a toddler, Lisa has been able to draw breath and consider her future more clearly. For first-time mothers, one of the inevitable questions (alongside when to return to work, when to stop breastfeeding, when to first leave the baby with a babysitter) is: should I have another child? This can be a challenging question for any woman but for an older mother it has added complications. Lisa has spent a lot of time contemplating the possibility of having another child. Now entering her forties, she knows that the biological clock is starting to tick even louder for her. The odds against conceiving are getting higher and the risk of miscarriage is also increasing. It's a lot to think about when you are trying to look after the child you already have and get your own life back together.

Definitely I would like to have another child but I would like to wait for my body to recover. The difficulty is that when you are older, the body needs more time to recover – but there is that pressure to have another child quickly. I would like to wait at least until Dexter is two and then try to get pregnant. I can't assume I will get pregnant – you just have to hope for the best.

In a perfect world, I would like to wait another five years, but I don't have the time. But I will wait as long as I can.

In the interim, Lisa intends to fully enjoy Dexter, who is now looking decidedly sleepy after polishing off most of his mother's cold peppermint tea. Or is that just wishful thinking on mum's part? He is still crawling into new frontiers – this time almost down the front step – as I prepare to leave. We decide to come down to Dexter's level and sit on the steps to wait for my taxi. We wouldn't have done that if Dexter wasn't around, but as Lisa had said earlier, everything changes when you have a baby. For older mothers, perhaps those changes are sometimes more acute.

Once you have had a baby the priority is to give it the best life you can. I think one of the things for me was that I was amazed by this little independent person and you just have to deliver them to the world as a good adult. That is my goal. And to keep my sanity. I don't think you realise how difficult that can be and it is worse when you haven't had any sleep.

One of the things that amazed me is how confronting and challenging being a mother is, on every single level. You change physically. Your brain isn't working when you are breastfeeding and you are trying to do your own work. You want to be a great writer and that has not changed, but at the same time you want to give this little thing everything you possibly can.

So for me the challenge is how do I do that? It is an opportunity to rethink yourself and rethink where you are headed over the next period of your life. And they just make you laugh.

For me, Dex is a gift. I don't know what I have done to deserve him, but nothing in my life has been better than this.

Marian Hudson

manager

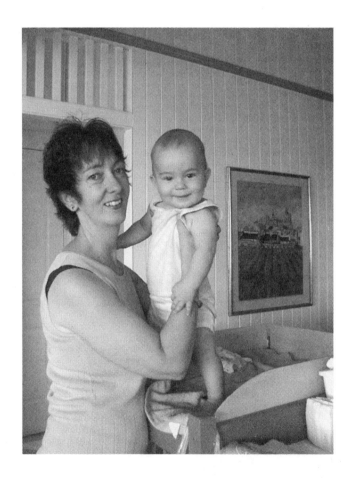

'I think I was caught up in that "have it all" era: that you could have a life, a job, a career; you could have everything and anything that you wanted . . . it never crossed my mind that I wouldn't be able to have a child.'

MARIAN HUDSON is in the kitchen of her Brisbane home joking about the kind of morning she has had. A 5.30am nappy change and breakfast for her baby son, Jack, was followed by an intense session of pureeing pears, an excursion to the laundry and, finally, breakfast for herself.

She makes it sound as if she is just a little fed up with this motherhood business and if you didn't know Marian or her recent past, you might be fooled into believing her. But Marian's self-deprecating humour is a cover. She doesn't mean to sound ticked off, not at all. Being at home with her seven-month-old son, Jack, watching him learning to crawl, doing his washing, mashing his food and getting up at dawn is fine by her. This time in her life, she says, looking at her son, is much too special to miss.

For Marian, 44, it is extra special because Jack is a surprise late baby. He was conceived just months after she and her husband, who has asked to remain anonymous, had given up all hope of having a family. Indeed, Marian had started retraining her mind and her heart to enjoy a life without children of her own. She would continue focusing on her busy and demanding job as a group manager for a major Queensland company.

Marian had come to this point after almost two and a half draining years of using IVF and other forms of assisted reproductive technology that had left her an emotional wreck after she failed to fall pregnant.

She was 42 when she finally decided she couldn't face another cycle of IVF. Marian knew that by this stage in her life there was only a very slim chance that she would fall pregnant by natural conception and, given her gynaecological history, had believed IVF was her only hope. It seemed to her that her failure to fall pregnant using IVF meant that her chances of conceiving were non-existent.

In a way, this was a relief as it meant she didn't have to keep hoping any more. As she was to tell me, in tears, it was the hope, followed by the disappointment of not having many successful egg pick-ups or embryo transfers, which had almost destroyed her during those years on IVF.

Up until this point in her life, Marian, a top-level group manager with Energex, one of the largest energy corporations in Australia, had succeeded at whatever she tried. In her career, which spanned more than twenty years working as a journalist, governmental press secretary and public affairs manager, she had gone from one successful job to the next. It had never crossed her mind that she wouldn't also be a success at motherhood. She had left marriage until later in life, but she didn't consider this a hindrance to her background plan to have children.

I didn't get married until I was nearly 37. I had delayed getting married because I had not met the right person. When we did get married, I wanted to have kids. Definitely. There was never any doubt in my mind about that. However, I waited.

I guess the thought never crossed my mind that I wouldn't be able to have them so I was in no hurry either.

I am quite embarrassed to say that I sort of knew that fertility fell off. But I didn't think about it and I didn't realise how much it fell off because in my whole upbringing no one ever said to me, 'By the way, if you want children you better have them before you are 35 or even 30, because your fertility goes down.' My conditioning was: you get married; you assume you have kids. That is what you were led to believe could happen and did happen, that kind of natural progression. Who out there is telling you that you can't have a child?

Indeed, nobody was saying loudly enough that the biological clock starts ticking faster in a woman's late thirties, eroding her fertility and making it harder for her to conceive. It's only been in the past decade or so that the issue has garnered attention in the media, and even then it has been dealt with in a political, rather than factual, manner. American Pulitzer Prize winning journalist Susan Faludi, in her 1991 book, *Backlash: The Undeclared War Against Women*, argued that much of the media reportage on a woman's ability to have children later in life was part of a conservative backlash against feminism and its fight to give women more choice. She cited a 1982 study published by the *New England Journal of Medicine* which showed that women between the ages of 31 and 35 stood nearly a 40 per cent chance of being infertile. 'This was unprecedented news indeed,' Faludi wrote, as 'virtually every study up until then had found that fertility didn't start truly declining until women reached at least their late thirties or even early forties.' Nevertheless, the *New York Times* put the news on the front page and the statistics made it into a number of alarmist books. However, as Faludi pointed out, the French researchers whose work was published by the *New England Journal of Medicine* had hardly used a representative group of women in their study. The women were all married to sterile men and were trying to get pregnant through artificial insemination.[1]

Society's mood regarding the dilemma of the biological clock versus women's right or need to a career was pretty much summed up by the economist Sylvia Ann Hewlett in her 2002 book, *Baby Hunger: The New Battle for Motherhood*. This book triggered an intense debate in the United States on the increasingly difficult juggle between wanting a career and finding the time and/or partner to have a child before a woman reached her forties and it was too late to start a family.

At the same time, the media continued to peddle 'miracle' stories about older women having babies, like the American singer Joni Mitchell, who had a baby in her fifties as a result of egg donation. The message from these stories was that with the help of assisted reproductive technology women could have it all at any age. It can be a shock, then, for many older professional women when they find out that they can't have babies to order. As Dr Stephen Steigrad of the Department of Reproductive Medicine at Sydney's Royal Hospital for Women said in a 2003 newspaper report, infertility will probably be the first major career disaster for many women in their thirties, who have worked hard for promotions and a nice home. This is a group, he said, not used to failing. Worse, it is their bodies that fail them and they can't fix it.

'They feel as though they are immortal, so why should they worry about kids?' he said. 'They are all out there getting themselves organised with the basics: two Beamers (BMWs), the garage, every whitegood creation, the plasma screen TV. They are saying: "We can't possibly have children yet." They have fought their way into some sort of career path and they may not have made a commitment to a partner until later in life.'[2]

Dr Steigrad was referring to the 'in control' generation, or those born in the early 1970s. Yet what he said is just as relevant to baby boomers like Marian, who was born into the generation that felt it was their right to make the most of the freedoms and opportunities available to them as a result of contraception, education and changing social attitudes. Educated at a private girls school, Marian was encouraged to achieve and succeed in her chosen occupation. This drive combined with the 'have it all' attitude of the 1980s and 1990s made Marian and many other women feel that it was okay to keep working hard to secure the house and the career and then think about having babies later.

I feel very strongly and quite angry now about this prevailing attitude that you can have it all. By the same token, you have to take responsibility for your actions. I think I was caught up in that 'have it all' era: that you could have a life, a job, a career; you could have everything and anything that you wanted.

I was caught up in that so it never crossed my mind that I wouldn't be able to have a child.

I don't know if I am a career woman; I think it just turned out that way, because I have never consciously planned a staged career. I have just enjoyed my jobs and done well at them and therefore progressed. So when you have that kind of success and ability to achieve you don't think, naively perhaps, that you can't have a baby.

A lot of my friends had babies at 37, 38 or 39 and they had them easily. I didn't know anyone on fertility treatments. My friends were having babies and I thought, 'Okay, I will have one now.' It was like I was hit by a semitrailer when I sat in the doctor's office and he told me that my chances of getting pregnant were 5 per cent.

Marian was then 40 years old. She had gone to see a gynae-cologist and obstetrician at a Brisbane fertility clinic. At that point Marian didn't even think she was infertile – she was just doing her research.

Being an organised, allegedly intelligent person who knew about things I decided it would be a good idea to see a specialist about having a baby at 40. I didn't go because there might be a problem. I just wanted to know about having a baby at 40. When he told me I only had a 5 per cent chance of conceiving I was gobsmacked. Absolutely gobsmacked. I had gone in there thinking I was doing my research. I was taking my folic acid and I simply wanted to know what else I needed to know.

Soon after seeing the specialist, Marian went on to an

assisted reproduction program, including IVF. After several months of trying to conceive naturally, she had failed to fall pregnant.

Over the next two and a half years, she was to have a veritable cocktail of treatments, including Timed Intercourse (TI), artificial insemination and IVF as well as frozen embryo transplants. Like any patient undergoing fertility treatment she was on a schedule of drugs to be taken orally, nasally, by injection or as pessaries inserted into the vagina. The drugs work according to the stages of the IVF cycle. To prompt ovulation, powerful hormone-stimulating drugs called gonadotropins are taken that will make a woman produce one or more eggs. The eggs are then 'picked up' – taken out of the follicles – at an egg retrieval. The eggs are then fertilised in the laboratory and put back into the uterus, which has been made more accommodating thanks to other drugs.

The egg retrieval usually requires a general anaesthetic. The transplant of a fertilised egg or embryo via a very fine catheter does not. Marian, however, had fallopian tube transfers, which do require a general anaesthetic.

The cost of Marian's IVF treatment came to about $15,000 after rebates from Medicare and her private health insurance.

It was an expensive journey, but the true cost was the emotional and physical toll of the treatments. Not usually a woman prone to tears, Marian can't hide her emotion when she starts talking about her years on IVF. You get the feeling that however much time passes, and despite the fact she now has a healthy young son, the pain she experienced will remain strongly in her memory.

The IVF experience was made harder because it didn't go

smoothly. In theory, the five-step IVF journey from ovulation to embryo transplant sounded straightforward, but in reality it proved complicated.

I was looked after by very good people and I had the best care, but my body just wouldn't co-operate. We would get to a cycle and then there would be no eggs to pick up or I would ovulate before we got to surgery. It was just difficult every step of the way. Quite often we didn't even get to the egg pick-up stage because there were no eggs to pick up or not enough to make it worth having the general anaesthetic.

The whole thing was the hardest thing I have ever done in my life.

The drugs made me teary. I was stressed. The drugs also gave me migraines like you wouldn't believe. I would spend two to three days in bed with the worst migraine, vomiting, and trying not to take headache drugs because I was worried about a pregnancy. Then I would get my period.

It was like going to a funeral every month. It was the worst kind of grief. Each month you would lose your dream of a family and then at the funeral you would have to decide that you were going to go back and do it all again – because I was up against a deadline given my age and didn't want to take the time out.

In the end I didn't know how to grieve. I can remember going to the hospital getting ready for an embryo transfer and I was about to go into theatre and they rang to say that all the embryos were abnormal. I just collapsed. My husband came and got me and I went home, changed into my work gear and went to work. I knew how to work but I didn't know how to cope with the loss.

The difficulties Marian was experiencing with IVF were exacerbated by the fact that few people knew she was having treatment. She had told close friends whom she could trust; however, she chose to tell only one person at work – her secretary. She had to, because the IVF treatment meant she went to hospital twice a month for procedures requiring a general anaesthetic. These commitments as well as the migraines and the emotional rollercoaster she was riding made work and IVF an almost intolerable mix.

She recalls how she ended up living a clandestine life with mystery appointments in her diary: 'You go to lots of meetings out of the office. It was like a covert operation when I was on IVF.'

During an IVF cycle Marian would go to the doctor at 7am several times a month for what she refers to as 'fan cam' – the intravaginal scans. She would self-inject egg-stimulating hormones and set her alarm for the middle of the night to drive to hospital for an egg-releasing injection prior to egg pick-up. She would then have to take a day off work for the egg pick-up, and then, two days later, take another two days off for the embryo transfer. All this, with trying to be 'normal' at work when all she wanted was to 'collapse with my own pain and grief', was difficult to say the least.

On occasions I caught myself yelling at people for no real reason and I realised it was my anger seething over and capturing some poor innocent victim in the cross-fire. Once I was in a meeting, the fearless leader negotiating some corporate deal or something and I had to go to the bathroom. To my horror I flushed another 'baby' down the toilet, burst into tears and nearly vomited.

I then had to return to the meeting and continue as normal. Another time I was holding a staff meeting and the reality of losing another chance at IVF hit me. I just collapsed on the desk and bawled my eyes out.

If it was so gut-wrenching, why continue with IVF? Logic, it seems, has little to do with it when the need to have a baby of your own is fierce.

I am stubborn and I wanted that baby so much. I think also when you are on IVF the cycle is a slow downward spiral. At the time I nearly lost my father and throughout it all I think I ended up not feeling. I stopped confronting my grief. I can remember on one occasion driving home and I was talking to a girlfriend saying, 'I am fine: I have just lost my babies but I am fine, and Dad's really sick, but I'm fine.' She said, 'I don't think you are dealing with it.' Then I collapsed in the biggest heap. I got so sick because I had internalised it all. I had switched off.

In an email message after our interview, Marian tried to explain further why she didn't stop IVF treatment, and why it was so important for her to continue even if the drugs were having such an impact and the disappointments were getting harder to bear. It was as if it was something she simply had to achieve no matter what the cost, financially or personally.

In my life I have achieved everything I have set out to, whatever the effort or application required, and I have had a good and fulfilling life. The baby was next on the list of things I wanted to 'achieve'. Failure is foreign to me so having a baby was in the same category and no one had ever told me I couldn't have a baby. I was going to have a baby and if I had to go through IVF and the associated trauma, sickness or whatever, I was going to do it at whatever cost. Every time I lost a 'baby' or the cycle 'failed' I just kept going, because giving up meant I would never have a child. Keeping going gave me some chance . . . until reality smacked me in the face. I was pushing shit uphill and for the first time in my life no matter how hard I tried or however committed I was, someone else was deciding this one. I had no control over the ultimate outcome.

After several unsuccessful cycles, Marian was described as having 'undiagnosed infertility', probably age-related. Even with high doses of drugs her ovaries had rarely produced more than one or two eggs. On only one occasion did Marian produce multiple eggs, but even they did not result in a pregnancy. She also fell pregnant once during IVF, however she miscarried very early in the pregnancy.

As hard as it was to live with the pain and disappointment she felt during IVF, it was even harder to stop.

It is the hardest thing to do because you are insane with grief and anger. I think it depends on the couple who feels it the most and how people deal with it in their own way. I just couldn't believe or understand what it could do to you, not just the drugs, but the disappointment – and I guess the drugs fuelling that. If someone had told me what it would be like I wouldn't have believed them – imagine losing a family member every month for two and a half years, imagine having to grieve in silence for someone you have lost. When I lost embryos or the cycle failed, I felt I had lost a baby or the chance of my own family. I just kept going because giving up meant I would never have a child.

One of the key frustrations for Marian during IVF was that she was not in control, that someone else was deciding her destiny. Finally, she couldn't take the stress any more and decided she needed to regain control of her life. She committed herself to three more attempts at embryo transfer, and to then using any frozen embryos that may be left. The first transfer was unsuccessful. For the second transfer, all three embryos were tested and found to be abnormal. She realised she simply couldn't face having another embryo transplant. The emotional pain had crushed any feelings of hope.

Marian again spoke to the specialist who had originally told her that she had a slim chance of getting pregnant by natural conception or by assisted fertility treatment. 'I remember saying to him, "I'm pushing shit uphill, aren't I?" He said "Yes, probably." I said, "I am not coming back."'

That was in April 2002. Despite her achievements and successes, Marian felt empty.

When it looked like I would remain childless my career seemed so hollow, although I have enjoyed all my jobs and worked hard at all of them. It seemed like all I had done in my life was point-less, although I had not consciously been working in preparation for a family. However, being part of the 'have it all' culture, I (in retrospect) had been gearing up to have a baby all my life; sort of like career, husband, house . . . oh and now it's time for the baby to magically appear. When it looked like a hollow dream I was devastated; sort of, 'Well now what am I supposed to do?' It all seemed so shallow and unimportant. It almost seemed like the universe was mocking me; some kind of sadistic payback for working so hard at my jobs and not breeding earlier!

Then, four months after Marian had decided to end IVF and begin accepting she would not become a mother, she fell pregnant. Jack was conceived in September 2002. When she found out she was pregnant, Marian 'went into absolute shock'.

I was starting to come to terms with never being a mum and then I thought, 'I don't know if I want this now.' I don't think this is what I really thought – I just didn't want to deal with so much emotional turmoil. I wanted the baby but I had started to get used to not having a family, and if I wasn't going to have a family, then I was going to enjoy my life.

My husband and I had started doing this and then I got pregnant. Then I thought I would lose the baby because I was pregnant once before during IVF and I lost it.

Then I thought after about two weeks that I am pregnant and I am having this baby. The same day I found out, I had written to my doctor to say thank you for his help; I never got a baby but I had the best help. I rang his receptionist and said, 'Did you get the letter? Well, throw it away, I'm pregnant.' She screamed down the phone and said, 'How did you do it?' I said, 'I tell you what, there wasn't a speculum in sight.'

Marian says everyone was on tenterhooks during her pregnancy, except her. She didn't worry despite the fact that this had been such a hard-won pregnancy. Somehow, Marian knew that it would be all right. However, it very nearly wasn't. She had decided to have an amniocentesis at 20 weeks.

I had a high chance of Down syndrome and many of the embryos before had gross chromosomal abnormalities so I just wanted to check him out. And I had a 1 in 250 chance of losing him through the amniocentesis.

The morning after the amniocentesis she awoke to feel liquid gushing into her bed – she was losing amniotic fluid. Everyone feared a miscarriage.

I knew what it was straightaway. I was just numb. I couldn't feel anything. I went to the doctor and then straight to the hospital but they can't do much really. You can only rest.

The resting worked and both mother and baby were okay, with Marian returning to work after two weeks. But there was more drama to come when Marian was diagnosed with gestational diabetes. This can cause health problems for the mother and the unborn child. So Marian had to go back to self-injecting, but this time it was insulin and not a fertility drug. 'By then I was used to needles,' she says.

Apart from these problems, Marian says she had a trouble-free pregnancy.

I had no morning sickness. It was wonderful. My doctor wrapped me in cotton wool. I thought having a Caesarean was the safest option. I am a small person and my sister had a difficult birth.

I didn't have a compelling urge to have a natural birth – I just
wanted to have a healthy baby.

Jack was born on 12 May 2003. It was November 2003
when we first met to talk about Marian's late baby, six months
after his birth, and the depth of her feeling for him was evident.
Jack is a beautiful boy with olive skin and brown eyes. The
next time we meet, a few weeks later, he has obviously grown
and is gallantly trying to crawl around the floor, often ending
up under the table. Marian reaches down to pull him out from
between its legs yet another time. She looks happy and relaxed.

I love being a mum. I went back to work for a little while after
Jack was born and while I like the mental stimulation and
I love the buzz that I get out of work, I love being with my baby
and I am going to find it extremely difficult to go back to work.

Marian is on a contract which allowed her seven weeks paid
maternity leave. She also had the option of taking a year's
unpaid leave. She had planned to return to work full-time in
September 2003, when Jack was almost four months old.

Initially, you could say that I thought I was superwoman. Old
habits are hard to break. I have to learn that I am not, and
relearn what is important in life.

She did go back for six weeks in mid-September when the
person who was filling in for her went on leave. Marian
describes those six weeks as 'terrible'. She says she has an understanding boss as well as an efficient staff section of up to six

people who report to her. Even so, she was putting pressure on herself to be the perfect mum and worker.

I couldn't cope with the stress of a challenging job and the demands of motherhood. It was self-imposed stress because I am a perfectionist and I was so concerned that I was tired and that I wouldn't be on the ball or have the energy I needed to deal with it. I love my job but juggling it with motherhood was very hard. My job is so deadline driven. If something happens you can't say I have to go home and breastfeed my son.

When we spoke, Marian was struggling with the dilemma that faces all mothers, older or younger: when to go back to work and what to do about that job if you find it incompatible with your desire to be a fully attentive mother to your child. This dilemma is often exacerbated for older mothers because we are talking about precious cargo. As Marian says, she and her husband tried so hard for Jack, and his care is something they both feel strongly about. By the same token, Marian acknowledges that her work also has its demands.

I think the reality is that in my position and at the level that I work, you either have to be full-time or find another job. And I don't expect charity from my employers. I expect them to be fair but they need to get the job done.

There is no doubt that having Jack has brought much fulfilment into Marian's life. Motherhood, she says, is better than she ever expected, despite the nights of broken sleep, the early mornings and the health hiccups which can seem terrifying to a new mum – but more often than not turn out to be ridiculously mundane. I ask her if Jack's happy presence in her home has helped her get over those traumatic years of trying for a baby through IVF.

I am not over it – I feel very strongly now about it. I encourage people to think about their fertility. People say to me you have got to get the house and they've got to get this and that. All this will happen – nothing else matters if you want a child.

It is also a mistake to think that if you are older and can't conceive naturally that you will go on IVF and have a baby. It's just not that easy. The media are keen to report all the 'miracle babies' conceived using fertility treatments, but they ignore the plight of the couples who remain childless despite the best medical teams and technology. Now I could name more than 50 women I know who are on IVF or some kind of fertility treatment. I don't know why this is the case. Perhaps we just lead more stressful lives. I can almost pick people who are on IVF now. I remember when I was walking around with my big fat belly, glowing, I felt awkward in front of people I knew who were on IVF and wanted a child. I was at pains to point out to them that my baby wasn't an easy conception.

Because Jack was a difficult conception and she is nearing her mid-forties, Marian accepts that he will be her only child. She says she finds it hard to be considered an older mother because she doesn't think of herself as old and never did – until she hit the fertility wall.

I always did things in my life when it suited me – I have never felt older. The first time was when I couldn't conceive.

As for having another child, I couldn't even go there right now. We never planned to have more than one child. Also, I just could not cope with the expectation of getting pregnant and losing it. I just couldn't. I thought I was a robust person until I tried IVF.

After hearing Marian's story of how hard it was for her on IVF it is a surprise to hear her also say that she would encourage any woman who is having trouble getting pregnant and who wants a child to try IVF. Her way of thinking is this: if you get to 50, and you still feel sad that you didn't have a child, you would not forgive yourself for not trying every avenue possible. Having Jack and knowing how wonderful it feels to have her son has made her even more adamant that if there is a chance to have a child, a woman needs to take it. Besides, there are many women who do not find the drugs problematic or who succeed in the first few cycles of IVF. It has helped thousands of women who would otherwise remain childless to achieve pregnancies.

However, Marian would caution women who were going on IVF that it is not a miracle cure for infertility in older women. Even so, she says women should be able to have the opportunity to try – and they should not have to try for a child in secret and then suffer in silence when they do not fall pregnant.

There is a silent epidemic out there that is impacting on so many people. There are so many women on fertility treatment or trying to have a baby and they, for whatever reasons – fear

*of career impact, their privacy, their embarrassment, the lack
of recognition as an acceptable medical condition – have to (or
choose to) deal with it alone, rarely with any broader support
than that which they get from close friends, family or the fertility clinics. (Mine was great and offered counselling which was
a godsend.)*

*Also, many women I know do not tell anyone and suffer
in silence without any outlet to air their fears or to get any
support. I chose to tell some people who were close to me as it
was easier to explain – 'Oh we can't come to dinner because
I will be in an operating theatre with a speculum shoved up
my twat and a truckload of strangers peering at my private
bits.' However, I was careful whom I told because I was so
emotionally fragile that I did not tell people who I thought
may be careless with my feelings. Then I was okay for people
to ask me how I was going, even if it resulted in tears – I still
needed people to ask me. If someone in the workplace had cancer
then they would be able to go openly to the hospital and have
treatment. They would also probably tell family, friends and
get some support. However, infertility is probably so much more
common yet women (and men) on treatment often feel they have
to sneak around and try to act as if nothing is wrong when
inside they are dying. People who have never been through
infertility will rarely be able to understand what it's like and
this is natural. But the ability of those seeking treatment to
cope with it is often undermined by the secrecy and the career
taboo it can be in some organisations. (Heaven forbid women
executives trying to have babies!) If it was understood and
in the open then I am sure it would be easier for those on it
to cope.*

Marian also says that women, especially older women, who are on IVF or other forms of assisted reproductive technology can be made to feel guilty or selfish for wanting a child and preparing to pay anything to get it. After all, these women have a career, a home and a husband – isn't that enough? As Marian or any woman who wants a child knows, yearning for a child is a different kind of want to the desire involved in looking at the plasma TV screens in a shopping catalogue. It is a deeply personal feeling that cuts to the core of who you are as a person. Having a baby later in life has only confirmed this for Marian.

You do get a lot of these guilt feelings – mainly you put it on yourself. It's like: in the global scheme of things I am lucky. I can't have a baby, but I suppose I should feel lucky. But you can't. I can remember someone said to me one day before I had Jack, 'Do you have children?' I said, 'No, I don't.' He said, 'You are lucky.' I turned back to him and said that I felt lucky about a lot of things in my life, but not about not having children.

For me, IVF was a living hell. I had counselling, I had the nicest doctors, but it was still hell. And many of the other women I know who are going through it feel the same way.

Now, I feel as if I have won Lotto. Now that I have Jack I know that everything I wanted and yearned for is real because he is all of those things.

Jacki MacDonald

former TV host, full-time mum

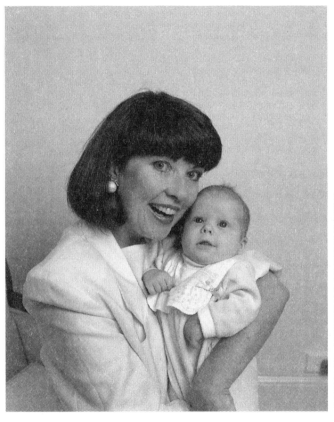

'My career was fabulous and I had never thought of kids. Because I had such a wonderful life, I would see people with babies with runny noses and sticky fingers and I just couldn't even see how that would ever be part of my life.'

YOU COULD SAY that the annual *TV Week* Logie Awards, television's 'night of nights', is an unlikely place to consider the prospect of motherhood. And it is true that Jacki MacDonald, then a popular small-screen personality and star of the variety show *Hey Hey It's Saturday*, even surprised herself when she spent most of the 1989 awards thinking of this very subject.

Of course, Jacki was no stranger to the event, having worked in the television industry since she was a teenager when she started reading the weather for Channel 9 in Brisbane. However, having babies was a completely alien concept. Up until then, Jacki was largely a stranger to any kind of maternal yearning. She jokes now that, when she was in her twenties, the mere sight of a drooling baby would make her maintain a promise to herself that she would never have anything to do with motherhood. And who had time for children, anyway?

Besides, by the time the 1989 Logies came around, she was still young enough, at 35, to wait a few more years before having children. Well, wasn't she? At least that's what Jacki told herself.

Those were the best of times for Australian television and Jacki was keen to make the most of it, as were her peers. She'd been in television for seventeen years by 1989, and had experienced great success. Private jets, lavish parties and a burgeoning collection of Logies on her mantelpiece were ample indication of her popularity.

They were heady days – this was the 1980s when the television networks were big spenders and only too happy to open their wallets for their stars and their publicity departments. Using private jets to whisk 'talent' to preferred destinations was part of the television whirlwind. It was, indeed, a fantastic career and one that Jacki embraced wholeheartedly. 'I loved it to death,' she says of her work during those days. 'We went to London for lunch and America for dinner.'

In 1989 there was no obvious reason for Jacki to stop loving it. Born in the central Queensland town of Blackall, Jacki had just won her fourteenth Logie. *Hey Hey It's Saturday*, which was about to celebrate its eighteenth birthday, was a ratings power-house and would continue to be so for Nine until it was axed in 1999.

Jacki had won the majority of her Logies in the category of most popular female personality in Queensland; however, her vivacious presence on *'Hey Hey'* had been noted by television executives always keen to find talent that attracts viewers. If Jacki wanted it, she could have had many more successful years in television.

And up until Christmas 1988 she had thought she wanted that kind of life. She was living in Brisbane and commuting to Melbourne to tape *Hey Hey* and had done so for eleven years. She played the publicity game well and often featured in magazines, although key events in her life, like her 1983 marriage to Brisbane skin specialist Dr Michael Pitney, were kept private.

But in May 1989, a few months after the Logie Awards, Jacki announced she was leaving *Hey Hey It's Saturday*. The reason? To have a family. Or, as she told *Hey Hey* host Daryl Somers on air during her last regular appearance on the show: 'If I don't give up now I'll never have any little owls. I'm an old duck.'[1]

At 35, Jacki wasn't what society generally refers to as an 'old duck'. She certainly didn't act old on television. In fact, her *Hey Hey* persona was youthfully zany. The media liked to call her 'wacky Jacki' and she was often photographed in hijinks mode – for example, wearing three birds on her head as a birthday bonnet when she returned to *Hey Hey* briefly to celebrate the show's eighteenth anniversary.

Jacki's madcap behaviour and easy laugh often deflected public comment on her age, and besides, even in the age-obsessed world of television, Jacki was relatively young. Even after she became a mother, she was still being offered jobs in her early forties. In 1991, in her late thirties, she had taken over from Graham Kennedy as host of *Australia's Funniest Home Video Show*.

However, the longevity of her television career was far from Jacki's mind when she quit *Hey Hey* in 1989. She was thinking instead of being a mother and knew she was at the age when fertility in women starts to fall. She acknowledged the prospect of missing out on having a family and wondered if she really felt all that averse to motherhood and drooling babies.

As Jacki says now, her career at the time was a huge distraction. There wasn't room for anything else in her life, apart from her husband and her pets.

Television liked to keep it that way. It can be an all-consuming medium, which demands absolute dedication and commitment from those who work in it – particularly those who wish to do well.

My career was fabulous and I had never thought of kids. Because I had such a wonderful life, I would see people with babies with runny noses and sticky fingers and I just couldn't even see how that would ever be part of my life.

And the industry didn't help, especially in the 1970s and 1980s. There was no room for that sort of thing. People weren't vaguely interested in people's children. You never even saw them.

So what caused her to stop thinking television and start seriously considering motherhood? Sitting in a Brisbane café, her tea going cold as she focuses on the question, Jacki recalls there were two key moments that made her rethink her life and her priorities. They made her consider two things. There was the inescapable reality that she was getting older and less fertile. And there was something else, something harder to define, a feeling that what she was doing – the constant commuting, the fast lifestyle – wasn't good for her physical or emotional health.

The first 'moment' came in the form of a friendly mental shove from her husband. There's a giggle from Jacki (some things never change) as she tells the story of how her husband caused her to tune in to her biological clock, and think babies rather than television ratings.

Michael and I had Christmas alone together one year – I was 35. He said to me, 'You women, you think you can have it all and in many ways you can have everything. But I am telling you that medical science says you cannot. If you have any intention of children you are really on the wire now. You either make a decision to keep going as you are or make the most of your last chance.'

Her response to her husband's words was typical Jacki Mac. She laughed. She still laughs today when she recalls the conversation.

But Michael's comments got under her skin, more than she originally realised. A few months later, in March, Jacki was at the 1989 Logies, sitting at the *Hey Hey It's Saturday* table, as usual, when Julie da Costa, Daryl Somers's wife, asked her a question.

She said to me: 'Are you thinking of having children?' I said, 'No, well, I'm not sure.' Everything was happening in front of me, but I was just sitting there thinking about what had just been said to me and how I had answered. I thought about it all the way home on the plane.

When she arrived home in Brisbane, Jacki thought more about Julie's question and her response. In fact, that's about all she could think about. Two months later, in May 1989, Jacki announced her surprise departure from *Hey Hey*. She had been a popular regular on the show for eleven years. There was no secrecy about why she was departing – she wanted to concentrate on starting a family. Considering Jacki's status and success in the TV industry, it was an unorthodox move. As *Hey Hey*'s executive producer, Gavan Disney, said at the time: 'She just wants to be Jacki Pitney. I admire her. She has had the guts to do what many wouldn't do – put family life before her TV career. She's turning her back on a lot of money and a lot of perks. She has told me she wants to have a baby. I'm sure that's what will happen.'[2]

Thirteen years later, Jacki remembers well how hard it was to give up her career, but at the same time she knew that she had no choice. Other women, she says, might have been able to cope with juggling the intense demands of television and motherhood, but she knew that she was not one of them. For her, the roles of motherhood and zany variety-show star were incompatible right from the beginning. Even before she fell pregnant she knew this. Having worked in television for almost two decades, she knew that it was a medium that doesn't make room for anything but work.

I decided that television and having a child were incompatible and that I couldn't do it publicly. I would have had to dress up as a duck or something like that on Hey Hey *and I thought, 'I don't want to do this', so I left.*

I left before I got pregnant otherwise I would have had to have gone through the whole discussion publicly. I didn't want to do it. I never did anything that meant a lot to me in public. When I got married to Michael it was a private ceremony. It was hard to decide about leaving television but I had just got to this point where I had no choice. I was either going to do that or that — and which was going to be the best for me?

Sitting there at the Logies was a very good thing for me. I thought, 'Am I really loving this or not?' and wondered how many more 'Hah hahs' I would have to do on Hey Hey *and when would they fire us from the show anyway? What would happen then? At the end of the day I just thought it was time to go.*

Looking back, Jacki says that in the late 1980s few, if any, high-profile women had been pregnant on television and she didn't feel like being a trailblazer. She is happy to see that now there are women who have managed to continue with their regular TV roles during their pregnancy, women such as Nicki Buckley, former *Sale of the Century* co-host, and ABC newsreader Juanita Phillips. *The Panel*'s Kate Langbroek even managed to breastfeed her baby on national television, an action which caused a remarkable amount of public debate with parties hotly divided over whether she should have done it or not. An older mother, Langbroek, who is in her late thirties, assumed, perhaps wrongly, that television viewers had more mature attitudes. Or maybe she was thinking of her child first and television second.

Jacki, however, had no intention of being pregnant in the intense glare of national television. So she did as she said she would — she quit and headed home to her large property on the western outskirts of Brisbane.

For a woman who had worked since she left school it was a strange new existence. Even stranger, perhaps, for someone who had lived in the public eye for so long and at such a heady pace. 'I felt a bit lost for six months and wandered around thinking, have I made the biggest mistake of my life?' Jacki says.

As for the matter of falling pregnant, Jacki says she didn't feel anxious. As it turned out, she had little trouble, and fell pregnant only a few months after leaving *Hey Hey*. Today, knowing how many older women struggle to fall pregnant either through natural conception or by using assisted reproductive technology, Jacki is surprised at how quickly she conceived.

> *It was amazing how I got pregnant so easily. I think it was because I thought I would. I just gave up on my appearance, went to the beach and lived a quiet life. There was always pressure in television – everything is an emergency.*

Jacki's first child, Lucy Kate, was born on 7 June 1990. Jacki was 36. She has since had two more children with Michael. Her son, Thomas, was born on 22 April 1993, and her second daughter, Emma Rose, was born on 26 April 1995.

Jacki was 41 when she had her third child. Now approaching 50, she says that she is grateful her husband alerted her to the ticking of her biological clock.

> *I was lucky he mentioned it because I would have kept going, as television is all-consuming. People just talk about what are we doing next year . . . you just roll along with it. I knew nothing about female fertility because it was something I wasn't particularly interested in. I was lucky because I got pregnant straightaway. And with the next two pregnancies I was very relaxed and I didn't care. If you care it can be harder, I think.*

Jacki's life is now focused on her three children and raising them to be happy, well-adjusted adults.

All I want is for my kids to be happy and get jobs that they love. They can do whatever they like as long as they are happy. They need a stable family life to do that.

These days she describes herself as a 100 per cent mother and she certainly seems relaxed in a role to which she is happy to dedicate all her time. Indeed, for a woman who didn't hold a baby until she cuddled Lucy in the maternity ward of a Brisbane hospital, Jacki has taken to motherhood with gusto.

I do everything around them and I don't think about any other thing. And it has made me very happy.

It wasn't always such a breeze and she remembers being in hospital in Brisbane after Lucy's birth and just staring at the bundle in her lap and wondering what on earth she was going to do with it.

It was like, 'Help me, I've been given a Martian.' When the nurse came in the following morning I had a pen and paper and I said, 'Now just tell me everything I need to know about how to run a baby.' I just didn't know the first thing about having a baby: what do they eat, how do I feed it. The nurse just looked at me and said, 'Rome wasn't built in a day.' After that we had a few days in the hospital to learn what to do, but there was always something different to learn with each child.

Jacki is hardly seen in the media these days and she is glad to admit that hers is a different world to the one still occupied by many of her friends in television. She relates how earlier that day she had been cleaning out the guttering of her home when she received a call from a close female friend – single, with no children – who had just returned from a holiday on Lake Como in Italy.

She loves her world and I love mine. That's just the way it is and we are both happy with where we are in our own worlds.

There have been times over the past thirteen years, however, when she tried to mix work with motherhood and returned to television part-time, at first after Lucy's birth and then after Thomas was born. She recalls how she worked on the *Midday Show* in 1994 when Derryn Hinch was host. Her job was to introduce new and ingenious products. She told the executive producer it would have to be a loose arrangement, and if her children fell ill she would have to stay at home with them and miss the show.

They said okay because I don't think they really thought about it. They think that you would never miss out on being on television because it is such a big deal, but in the end it is not a big deal when you have children and they are sick.

I had to call one day when the kids were sick and said, 'Hello, I am not coming because one of my kids has got a temperature.' They said, 'What! You've got to be joking!' I said, 'No, unfortunately not, so we will talk again next week.' I was a bit disappointed and I started to realise that the two things were incompatible. You can't do the two things at once when you have young children. There is always going to be something that suffers. One of the executive producers on the show said to me she knew how I felt. She said she put her child in a crèche at 7am in the morning and then she cried all the way to work. I said you're mad, you should tell these people to get lost.

Jacki didn't exactly tell the television industry to get lost, but after working on several post-*Hey Hey* jobs, including *Australia's Funniest Home Video Show*, the *Midday Show, Healthy, Wealthy & Wise, Brisbane Extra* and a position with Foxtel, she decided she would not return to television after the birth of her third child, Emma.

Eight years later she has maintained that decision. She has opted for a low-key life, preferring to sort out school projects and organise family holidays rather than re-enter the razzle-dazzle of television. It's been years since she posed for a photo-shoot, though there was a time when a reader couldn't open a women's magazine without coming across a story on Jacki Mac. She says she hasn't spoken to any of the magazines for ages and doesn't care to either. A shame, as she would still make good copy.

The day we meet Jacki is dressed in a white linen pantsuit. She wears no make-up except pink lipstick. She is as ebullient and vivacious as she was on television and appears to have changed little since those madcap days. So much so that you almost expect her *Hey Hey* offsider Plucka Duck to turn up for coffee as well. Jacki was always anything but self-conscious – how else do you keep smiling while picking up frozen fowls in 'Chook Lotto' week after week? It's no surprise then to see her whip out her pink nail polish at the café table to do a quick touch-up while waiting for her tea to arrive.

The self-imposed media silence is no deep mystery, she says – she is simply too busy being a mother. She chooses not to do publicity just as she chooses not to work full-time in television or in any other job while her children are young.

Jacki has been able to make this choice because she is a canny businesswoman. Even when she was working on *Hey Hey* and being paid well for her weekly hijinks by the Nine Network, she had other business interests. During the 1980s she was a director and partner in a Brisbane-based production company and also had her own floral business. She has long since sold her shares in these companies, but maintains an avid interest in real estate which she has pursued since the 1980s.

Jacki has always been particularly savvy about real estate, and dealing in property has brought her both pleasure and wealth. In 1995 she told the *Australian Women's Weekly* that she used her spare time when the children were napping to buy and sell real estate.

I like real estate. It's a gut instinct thing. I buy and renovate things for myself, which means I earn enough money to do the things I want to do. Women should always have something they are doing for themselves to earn money, because you never know what is going to happen in your life.[3]

Almost nine years after that interview, Jacki says her decision to give up working in television to focus on motherhood was made easier by the fact that she could financially survive without *Hey Hey It's Saturday*.

I was lucky but then I had worked hard and I had always loved real estate. For all of those years that I had been working in television I had invested elsewhere because I knew that television was not for ever. None of those careers are. They are dependent on whether people like you and people are fickle.

The mother of two daughters, Jacki is well aware that one day her own children will have to face the same sorts of decisions she did fifteen years ago, when it became evident to her that if she was going to have children she needed to act, and that there was the distinct possibility motherhood would clash with her career. What would she say to her daughters about these decisions they may face?

I think everybody gets to have children when they are really ready. I think mothers who have their babies early have other things to offer. They can run faster than me. Older mothers have had the opportunity to have a career, to put all their energy into their lives and their career. I have to say it is hard having a career – I couldn't do it now.

I never really thought about my age when I had children because all my friends now are a lot older than me. They never seem to have obstacles that they can't get over. I am lucky to have these guys as role models so I would never be game to say anything like this is hard. I am just a young pup. I don't think age has any drawbacks at all when you are a mother. The only thing I was worried about was that I was so cumbersome when I was pregnant. But I love having children. They are the most divine people.

Jacki laughs at how her life looks like coming full circle,

with her youngest daughter, Emma, asking to go to boarding school. Jacki, who was born on a cattle and sheep property, was sent to boarding school between the ages of ten and eighteen. She recounts how her independent eight-year-old daughter has suggested she should also go to Jacki's former school, New England Girls School in Armidale, New South Wales.

Not because of me but because she can take her horse. My mother says Emma is not like me when I was eight because I was polite. She is more like me as I am now.

Jacki's devotion to her children looks like it came at the cost of her career. However she doesn't see it that way. Instead, she sees her departure from television as the beginning of another brilliant career – as a mother. Just as she took affirmative action and decided she had to stop her working life to focus on children, she ultimately made the decision to choose motherhood over continuing in television. In many ways, this was because she was an older mother – she knew how precious her children were. Also, she had the financial ability to make this choice. And she had a strong and secure relationship with her husband. All of this came about over time. For those mothers who have to divide work with motherhood, Jacki's seems a fortunate life and an enviable one.

She is lucky and she knows it, as do other contemporaries who are older with children. She tells of one of her former *Hey Hey* cohorts, saxophonist Wilbur Wilde, who has become an older father of twins.

He is so excited about it and I think that is the thing about

*having children when you are older. You do just feel so lucky.
When you are young you expect it. When you are older you just
feel lucky because you appreciate that you really have run the
risk of not having them.*

*Most of my friends don't have children and they have
fabulous lives without them. But I am just one of those people
who has loved it.*

I wouldn't be surprised if Jacki told me she didn't even
watch television these days. Being a mother is much more
interesting and fulfilling. Ironically, though, for all its shallow-
ness, it was television which gave Jacki deeper insight into
what sort of older mother she wanted to be.

*I had a great childhood. My mother was always there. I was
living in the country and then I went to boarding school but
I always came home to the country. The moments in television
that were very difficult and I was in a hotel room on my own,
I would think about that time when I was a kid. I want my
kids to have that, to remember their childhood as a time of fun
and happiness because you need it for the rest of your life.*

Lisa Bolte

former principal artist,
the Australian Ballet; full-time mum

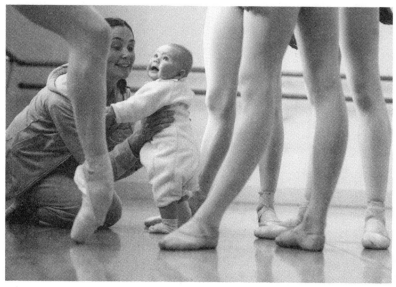

'When I was dancing I thought I had to be there 100 per cent or it wouldn't work . . . I can't imagine having devoted myself to a baby as well during this time.'

FOR FIRST-TIME MUM and former ballerina Lisa Bolte, one of the enduring images of her daughter Olivia's first year was watching her take her first steps. She was delighted to have her own parents with her to share this pivotal moment in their granddaughter's life. As Lisa looked on, she knew her daughter's achievement had taken determination. In her own life, including her sixteen-year career as a ballerina, she'd had to learn many new steps too, both on stage and off, in order to succeed. Lisa was to learn that this wasn't going to change after she left the Australian Ballet in 2002 when she gave birth to Olivia.

When I first approached Lisa about being involved in this book it was partly out of curiosity. What was it like to experience such a dramatic change from being an intensely focused dancer who travelled the world with a ballet company that was like a family to her, to being a retired ballerina and first-time mother at 35? I had seen Lisa dance on many occasions with the Australian Ballet, both in Melbourne, where the company is based, and in my home town of Brisbane, where it tours annually. Her career was of particular interest to me as I had danced as a child through to my teenage years and I knew full well the dedication needed to get to the top of this demanding profession. Also, although Lisa was born in Sydney, she had started her dancing lessons in Brisbane and was considered a 'local' by the Queensland dance fraternity.

She was initially happy to be involved in the book and keen to tell her own story about being an older mum. However, a few months later I spoke to her again, and she was unsure if she should be part of the project. This was because the complexion of her life had changed dramatically since our first conversation.

Lisa had separated from her fiancé, Olivia's father, when Olivia was eight months old and she didn't want her story of motherhood to sound negative. I suggested it wouldn't be, but might instead be familiar to many women, older and younger, who have found themselves alone after the birth of their child as a result of a relationship breakdown.

Unfortunately this can be the unhappy flipside of having a baby, with the stresses involved in becoming a parent some-times causing fissures in a relationship to crack wide open. Lisa knew this. She also knew she wasn't the only woman to find herself alone with a new baby. Nor was she trying to hide it.

However, as it turned out, the positive experiences of first-time motherhood made Lisa decide to go ahead and tell her story. She had learned many powerful lessons and she wanted others to know that being a mother, albeit a single mother, at 37, was something which she did not regret. Not at all.

When Lisa was a leading ballet dancer, there were always new roles to discover, contemporary works to explore, different interpretations of the classics and countless strange stages around the world which, out of necessity, needed to become instantly familiar. Even as a child dancing in a suburban ballet school in Brisbane, Lisa was keen to soak up as much information as she could and use it to perfect her dancing. It was this attitude which was later to help her progress through the ranks of the Australian Ballet, becoming a principal dancer at the age of 27.

For the past year or so her determination and positive attitude to life has helped her cope with her new role as a mother to Olivia, who was born in November 2002. A few months earlier she had retired from the Australian Ballet, where she had been a company member for sixteen years, to concentrate on being a full-time mother.

Since then, she has taken to motherhood with the same grace which always set her apart as a dancer. Still, like any role worthy of a prima ballerina, there have been some challenges. The biggest challenge has been the break-up with her fiancé, whom she wishes not to name.

As with any break-up, there have been tensions and the past year has been traumatic and bewildering for Lisa, who never imagined she would experience the end of her relationship, especially with a child involved. Lisa tries not to dwell on the negatives, and instead finds comfort in the fact that she has a healthy and happy child in Olivia.

I really feel this is the right time for me to be a mother. To me, that is one of the things about being an older mother. I have had this amazing career and danced in many fantastic places around the world. I have had beautiful partners in dance. I can still walk in to the Australian Ballet and feel like family there.

I don't feel as if I have had to make sacrifices to be a mother. I feel as if I sacrificed my own family more in doing ballet. Just the fact that I have had twenty years of living away from them. Despite that we are very close.

I have had four months with Olivia with Mum and Dad and it has been one of the most special times in my life. Mum and Dad were there when Olivia walked and to see the excitement on their faces . . . it was wonderful. She is their first grandchild and it has been amazing for all of us. I find it very hard to be apart from my family now.

Since she was a seven-year-old child, ballet has been an enduring passion for Lisa. She remembers it was at this age that she learned of the famous English ballet dancer Margot Fonteyn, who had formed one of the world's classic dance partnerships with Russian star Rudolf Nureyev. During the 1960s they were the Richard Burton and Elizabeth Taylor of the dance world, feted by the media and jetsetting to famous stages around the world.

In 2002, on the eve of her retirement, Lisa recalled that people had remarked on Fonteyn's beauty and radiance, and these words had affected her deeply and stayed with the young dancer throughout her career.[1]

Fonteyn was a wonderful role model for a young dancer. An exquisite ballerina, the British dancer dedicated herself to her career, performing until she was 60. She died at the age of 72 in 1991. Lisa remarks that one of the reasons she left it until her mid-thirties to start thinking about having children was that her lifelong role models had been ballerinas like Fonteyn who did not have children. Their passion was for dance. Lisa wanted more than anything to be like Fonteyn, which meant absolute dedication to her profession from a young age.

> *Because I had a career that seemed to keep going until later in my life, I didn't even think about having children. I just wanted to be a ballet dancer. That is all I ever wanted to do. I was really passionate about it from a young age. Children never fitted into the picture at all. I used to read ballet books and a lot of the ballerinas who were my role models never had children. Dancing was a way of life for these women. So I never associated myself with having children until I was about 33.*

It's not hard to work out why famous ballerinas like Fonteyn did not have children. Classical ballet is a hard taskmaster. If a dancer is not busy doing class, she is rehearsing for a new season or touring. Inevitably, the ballet company becomes like a substitute family and this is where a dancer looks for friendship and comfort. There is little time in a dancer's life for relationships outside the company in which she is a member. Certainly, for a young dancer hoping to be promoted through the ranks of a ballet company, there would be no room for too many other grand passions.

Lisa was one of those dancers with a passion, having joined the Australian Ballet School at sixteen. She was accepted into the Australian Ballet in 1986 and quickly rose through the ranks, coached by (former) artistic director, Maina Gielgud, who cast Lisa in principal roles after only a year with the company. At 20, Lisa was already learning some of the most demanding roles in the classical repertoire, including Aurora in *The Sleeping Beauty*. It was after dancing this role at the prestigious Royal Opera House in Covent Garden, London, that Lisa was promoted to soloist in 1988 at the age of 21.

It was a stunning achievement for Lisa, who proved she had the passion to work hard. Five years later she was promoted to principal, the highest level for a dancer in a ballet company.

Despite her success, Lisa knew that there was usually only a small window in life, maybe through to her mid-thirties, when a woman can dance the key classical roles. And that this window could very easily be closed due to injury. If she wanted to be a principal ballerina the need to focus on dance was paramount.

It can be such a short career in ballet, and I think, for me, I never was quite sure I would have the physique to go back to ballet after I had a child. For most of my career being a ballet dancer took all of my drive. When I was dancing I thought I had to be there 100 per cent or it wouldn't work. When I came home from ballet, I would watch videos and read information and books [about ballet]. I can't imagine having devoted myself to a baby as well during this time.

Also, Lisa had looked around her and seen how great a commitment it was for a female dancer to find time outside ballet to have a family. It's tough for any leading dancer, but according to Lisa it is particularly difficult for dancers in the Australian Ballet, a small, hard-working company committed to touring several months of the year. Throughout her career she was away from her Melbourne base for up to eight months each year. Under these circumstances, it was virtually impossible for her to even consider having children in her twenties.

Besides, her heart wasn't in it as ballet was her passion. Also, Lisa knew from her own personal experience of working with leading ballet dancers who also had children that this was not an easy combination. It took resolve and a particular kind of determination. So particular it seems that there are no dancing mums in the Australian Ballet. There are only two parents in the main company – and they are men, principal dancers Steven Heathcote, who has two children, and Campbell McKenzie, who has one child.

It is very hard in this demanding schedule in a ballet company to have children. A few people have managed it, such as Marilyn Rowe [former Australian Ballet principal] and Marilyn Jones [also a former principal]. But you need to have the right circumstances for it to work. Another dancer, Paula Baird, who was a soloist with the Australian Ballet, managed to continue with her career because she had an auntie who helped look after her child and travelled with her when she went on tour with the company. Family support is crucial in this instance.

In the late 1990s, Lisa's career was still going strong. She had performed in the United States, China, Canada and across Europe, and danced most of the classical repertoire, including crowd favourites such as *Giselle* and *Swan Lake*. Choreographers had created works for her, with Lisa proving herself adept at both contemporary and classical dance. She had also won scholarships, which had taken her around the world studying dance. There had been some hiccups as a result of injury. Stress fractures in her feet had caused her major problems. Even so, she was still a beautiful dancer when she announced, at 35, that she was retiring from the Australian Ballet. So what prompted this change of heart from a woman whose life, up to this point, had been dedicated to dance?

> *I thought I had met the right person. And, I suppose, that is when you start to think about children. You also start to see your parents who are longing for grandchildren, and I didn't want to leave it too late. Also, I was reading things in the newspapers about leaving it too late and it was starting to worry me. I didn't know that much about it but I had always thought, well, if I have children before I am 40 then that's okay. Then gradually I came to want children more and more. I also didn't want to be a too much older mum.*
>
> *My mum had me when she was 22. I can remember having the perfect childhood. I had a young mum who had so much energy for her children. I wanted to be like that.*

Lisa and her partner had been together for four years and engaged for three and a half years. When Lisa decided the time was right for her to try to have children, she had little trouble falling pregnant.

By the time she announced her retirement in April 2002, she was already four months pregnant. She was still dancing, but it had been a tough first trimester. When she was six weeks pregnant she had a health scare. Doctors told her there was a chance she could lose the baby. The baby's heartbeat was slow and Lisa was told to rest. She followed instructions, and returned to the stage once the problem was rectified, confining herself to roles that she felt were gentler on her body.

She also suffered terribly from morning sickness and was forced to stop doing classes at the Australian Ballet. Her body couldn't handle the physical work and she remembers having to leave class to be sick. She also remembers the only time she didn't feel sick was when she was performing, which was a godsend as she was still in demand as a principal dancer with the company. Being on stage somehow took her into another realm where there was no nausea – only that familiar feeling of strength and fulfilment.

When Lisa stopped dancing altogether, her morning sickness stopped as well. But how hard was it to make that decision to retire? Lisa knew that she could not manage the juggle of dance and a newborn baby, and yet it was hard to leave the Australian Ballet.

I was in two minds about it. I didn't know whether or not to leave the company. I still had a lot of love for dance but I felt I had left it until now to have a baby and I wanted that baby to be my first priority. I wasn't sure if I could go back and be totally committed to dance. I thought I could go back and do some guesting and see what happened further down the track.

When I stopped dancing, healthwise I didn't look back. I didn't have any more morning sickness. I felt great. I had a long birth – a 24-hour labour. I went into hospital at 5pm on a Saturday and Olivia was born at 5pm the next day. It was 3 November 2002.

Immediately after Olivia was born, Lisa knew she had made

the right decision about leaving dance, even if it meant it would be harder for her to return to ballet if she wanted to when she was older. She was determined to concentrate on being a mother to Olivia and she knew that without family support in Melbourne (her parents live in northern New South Wales), it would be hard for her to combine dancing and motherhood.

There were other concerns in Lisa's life at that time, more pressing than combining motherhood with classical ballet. Problems in her relationship with her fiancé were intensifying.

They had planned to marry. But after Olivia was born the tenor of the relationship changed. Lisa made herself face the sad fact that it wasn't working and the couple split up in July 2003.

Lisa felt she needed to be near loved ones and went to stay with her parents. She has since returned to Melbourne where she lives in a flat with Olivia. Her former partner has access to Olivia, though at the time of writing a more formal arrangement was yet to be decided.

This sudden change of circumstances in her life caused Lisa great pain. She felt as if she was on an emotional rollercoaster, having left the ballet company she'd been part of for sixteen years and become a new mum only to have her relationship with Olivia's father end in tears.

I feel very sad that it hasn't worked out. You don't go into a relationship lightly. When you have a baby it is a very fragile time. I want my daughter to grow up in a happy environment. I felt as if I had no choice but to leave the relationship.

I don't think how old you are matters when this happens to you. I think it would be terrible at any age. A break-up is a shocking thing. Having a break-up without children is terrible. When children are involved it is even more distressing because you worry about the child's future.

I found it really difficult to leave [my partner]. My parents have been together for 38 years and I always saw my relationship also having a long life.

You never can tell the way life is going to go. My only regret is that I was not strong enough to keep my independence in the relationship.

Women of any age, older or younger, who are going into a relationship should be careful and protect themselves in all ways, financially and emotionally. They should think carefully about their careers. They should be wary about signing their lives away.

For me, I will have to see what happens. Lots of good things come to good people and I believe it will work out. I don't have any regrets about having Olivia. She is the most beautiful thing to happen to me in my life. I have had many amazing things happen to me; I have great friends and family. This little girl has surpassed everything.

She brings such joy and I am sure that is what children do. That's what makes the world go round.

Lisa's joy in having Olivia has made her consider her own upbringing and how different her life has been compared to that of her mother. She remembers having a wonderful childhood with her younger siblings, two sisters and a brother. Now, having had Olivia, Lisa finds it somewhat sobering to realise that her mother had four children by the time she was 24. And the last two were twins.

By the same token, Lisa's parents were of a different generation – her mother looked after the children (a job which
included driving Lisa and her siblings to the local ballet school)
as well as helping in the family landscaping business. Her
father worked full-time as an environmental scientist. Lisa says
her mother is one of the most inspiring people she knows, but
she acknowledges that becoming a mother in her twenties
would not have suited her.

*Now, after having Olivia, I can't imagine being a younger
mother, because I had this yearning to be a ballet dancer. You
don't think about anything else – it is this vision. I feel that
being an older mother has been good for me. It wasn't that I
didn't think having children younger was impossible – I never
saw Mum not coping with life or out of sorts. She is such a well-
balanced lady and it has always been that way. I have an added
respect for her and I think many other women feel the same way
about their mothers after they have had children.*

*Now I know that I was lucky to be able to put all that energy
into myself for a long time. Ballet is quite a self-centred career.
If you are not focused on your work you will not make it. By
24, Mum had four of us. I am 37 and by the time Mum was
37 I had left home to go to the Australian Ballet School. I try
now to imagine how it must have been for her to have her little
girl leave home then.*

Initially, Lisa wanted to leave the Australian Ballet to devote
herself to Olivia. Even so, she never pledged full retirement. In
2002 she appeared in a guest 'character' role as Lady Capulet
in the company's production of *Romeo and Juliet*. She had to ask

friends to look after Olivia during rehearsals and performances. It was a juggle but she managed. She says the experience made her realise that she hadn't fully given up the idea of going back to dance.

Despite her love for Olivia she couldn't quite discard her passion for dance. And why should she? The times are changing in regard to the acceptance of older dancers and there is a new breed of ballerinas who are determined to combine motherhood with a longer career in dance.

One of these women is Britain's Darcey Bussell, who could easily be a new kind of role model for budding ballerinas. She is an exquisite dancer, but unlike Fonteyn, this dazzling star of the Royal Ballet married young and had her first child at the age of 31. She returned to dance about six months later and undertook a gruelling tour of Australia, bringing her one-year-old baby, Phoebe, who was teething at the time, with her. That didn't stop Bussell dancing the lead role in *Swan Lake*. She seemed to take it all in her stride and was even spotted doing some shopping at Woolworths during the Royal Ballet's Brisbane season.

Late in 2003 she took another break from dance to have her second child. Zoe Sophia was born in February 2004. A ballet megastar in the United Kingdom, Bussell knows that she is a valued member of the Royal Ballet and the company would do anything to keep her happy. As a result, she has excellent support from the company to help her balance her job with being a mother. Not many other dancers would be in such an enviable position. Certainly, Lisa says that for her to go back to dancing full-time she would need to be offered the right roles and would also need a lot of very good support.

This might be difficult, she says, as she has no family in Melbourne. Also, she wants to spend as much time as she can with Olivia while she is young.

I am loving this stage in my life with her. Why go and spoil that time? It is so precious. I think she is really thriving because I am there all the time. She has hardly had any time away from me. She is a very happy little girl and she has had constant contact with her mother since she was a baby. I am not in a rush to change this.

Even so, financial pressures are a serious concern. The break-up with her partner forced Lisa to give up the part-time work she enjoyed as a teacher at the Australian Ballet School, which she had started when Olivia was a few months old. Now she only works sporadically when she can get friends or family members to look after Olivia, as she cannot afford to pay for care.

I had work which I loved and I had to give it up because I am now the primary carer of Olivia. I was working with the Australian Ballet School teaching the graduate year of students which I really enjoyed because they have a passion for dance.

My priority now is to sort through what is happening in my life. The hard thing is that I don't have any family here in Melbourne and that is part of the reason why I can't work. Olivia is too young, she needs her mother at the moment so that is my major role and it will be that way until she gets older. To be honest, I am uncertain what my future work will be. For the time being I just have to wait and see.

With so many parts of her life in flux, Lisa says she feels as if she is in limbo — an unfamiliar sensation for someone who has had such purpose in her life for so long. She says she doesn't know what the future holds in regard to many facets of her life. Despite the fact that she is unhappy about some elements of her life, she feels positive about others. She is physically fit after having Olivia and believes that if called on, her ability to dance would return. It would take some hard work and dedication, but Lisa is no stranger to either. 'I think you can do anything if you set your mind to it,' she says.

She says she doesn't feel at all disadvantaged by her age, reiterating that she chose the right time in her life to have Olivia. At 37, she says she can look back on an amazing career of dance and look forward to a life with her child — and, if things work out, maybe another chance to dance. If she had it her way, this future would include having another baby.

I would have another child tomorrow, just like that. I love children and I love being a mother. Maybe that is the body clock talking! I have had such a special time with Olivia that I would love to see her with a little brother or sister. But I have to count my blessings. We will just have to wait and see what happens.

Claudia Keech

*international publicist,
founder of motherInc*

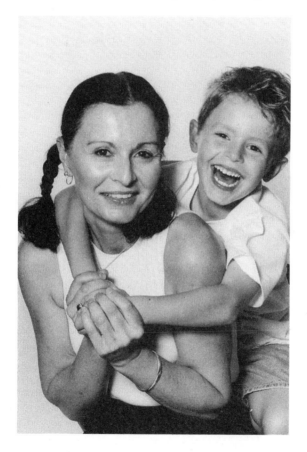

'I always thought if I was able, I would love to have a child. I wasn't consciously letting it slide.'

HAVING A BABY — at any time in life — can have a profound effect on a woman, the new arrival sending shock waves through her attitude to her work, her relationships and all other aspects of her life. For older, professional women, in particular, juggling the demands of child, partner and work can lead to a reassessment of how they are going about their lives and what they can do to change them.

Claudia Keech, a one-time international publicist, founder of the website www.motherinc.com.au (motherInc) and a first-time mother in her forties, is one of those women.

Two years ago Claudia sat down to peruse the results of a poll on maternity leave carried out by her popular website for modern mothers. The woman who had introduced Americans to the delights of Australian tourism, Foster's lager and the art of Ken Done in the 1980s would not have been too surprised by the responses of more than 1000 women. They gave over-whelming support to the concept of three months maternity leave on full pay, to be funded by the federal government.

Nine years ago, Claudia had her own experience of maternity leave – make that her former employer's concept of maternity leave. In 1995, then in her early forties, she gave birth to Callan.

Before his birth she had been working overtime – which was fairly typical for this high-energy woman – on a project for magazine publisher Time Inc, promoting its new magazine, *Who Weekly* (now *Who*). She spent three months training some-one to do her job so that she could take six weeks off with her new baby, without too much interruption, she hoped. The plan was to then work primarily from home for another few months. Little did she know that she would start work again soon after Callan's birth – from her hospital bed.

I got a phone call within 24 hours of giving birth in the hospital. I was on pethidine and still can't remember what I said, but it must have been the right answer at the time! Now I can laugh at that phone call, but looking back I sometimes wonder whether I should have just called in with food poisoning to secure at least 24 hours off duty.

Claudia tells this story with typical candour and good humour. She knows the ropes of the media business better than most, and it was just one of the crazy things that has happened to her over the past twenty years as a journalist and publicist. In retrospect, though, she considers it a timely wake-up call – life for this older mum, sooner or later, had to change.

And it did. Claudia's story is telling, as it shows how having a baby later in life can become a tool for change – and how being older and wiser helped her take the first crucial steps.

Three years ago, Claudia's professional and personal life merged when she channelled all her knowledge and media savvy into starting a website for mothers. She remembers how she was standing at the gate of her son's preschool one day and realised that every other mum was just like her – stressed and rushed off her feet.

We were all the same. Stressed and time-poor. We were trying to juggle work and family with not a lot of time for ourselves.

She did her research and decided motherInc would be an online resource for the savvy modern mother, offering support and guidance on social issues as well as information on new products. Three years since it was launched in 2001, mother-Inc has more than 100,000 subscribers and has developed into a credible resource for businesses and governments needing to know what's on the mind of the twenty-first-century mum.

The website is a success, but it never would have happened if Claudia hadn't given birth to Callan. For Claudia, becoming a mother late in life has changed just about every aspect of her life. It eventually led her to turn her back on the corporate world and set up a home business. However, after almost three years of running motherInc on her own, Claudia has decided to merge her business with a publisher and has had discussions with major publishers in Australia and the United States. She is hoping such a new relationship will lead to motherInc having a global impact. Claudia says it was time for a change. The website has grown from a support and information resource to a seriously popular on-line magazine for women and mums, and there was too much work involved to keep it 'in house'. This move will take some of the pressure off Claudia and her decision to merge with a publisher is another example of how she has shaped her life according to her needs. She has made the most of opportunities and says that in many ways her mature age has helped her recognise when change is needed – especially in that titanic struggle of trying to maintain a job, a marriage and a relationship with your children. However it hasn't always been easy.

As well as being a new mum working in demanding jobs in the media, for a few years, before she met her third husband, Michael Harris, Claudia was a single mother.

Just like many older women to whom I have spoken for this book, Claudia thought that she would never become a mother. Hers is a common refrain in that she was too busy working in her twenties and thirties to give the subject of children much thought. But there was an additional reason for her hesitation. She believed her hopes of motherhood had been dashed forever after she suffered a miscarriage in her late thirties.

This was hard to bear, as Claudia had finally met the man she thought was perfect for her. Yet just as her heart had found the right mate, it seemed as if her body was going to let her down. By then she was nearing forty, but had never considered herself 'old'.

For me, when I was in my twenties and thirties, it was a case of feeling so young in many respects . . . it was not like I wasn't going to have a child or that I was even consciously leaving it late. I was just getting on with having a great life and a great career. I always thought if I was able, I would love to have a child. I wasn't consciously letting it slide. I suppose it ended up late for the obvious reasons – I was travelling the world and having a fabulous life and my past did not take me towards being in a committed relationship with children. My brain just wasn't there. I used to say to people after Callan was born that I should be wearing that T-shirt that said I forgot to do something – have a baby. It was never not the plan and it was something that would be really terrific to do – later on.

Claudia says she was 'full throttle' into her career during her twenties and thirties, but you get the feeling this is a woman who hardly ever has her foot off the accelerator. We arranged our meeting to talk about late motherhood at a café in Milsons Point Sydney, as Claudia planned to squeeze in a few laps at the nearby North Sydney Pool. As well as keeping up a busy work regimen, she likes to exercise regularly. The pace doesn't let up at night – it's not unusual for Claudia, after a full day's work, to be sitting at a computer after her son has gone to bed working on her own projects or a project for Callan's class at school.

She has always been a bit of a workaholic, starting her career in the media in Western Australia where she began a glossy magazine called *Girl About Town*. Advertisers immediately embraced it so Claudia and her co-founders decided to take advantage of the situation and sell the rights to the magazine. It was renamed *Our Town* and Claudia stayed on as a journalist.

I worked like a demon. I am one of those people who says, 'Well, why not, let's do it!' I had been to America for stories for the magazine and I thought a lot of American products come to Australia, but we have so many great things here that could do well in the US. I didn't have import skills but I could do PR.

Claudia took a chance and relocated to Los Angeles where she started her own international public relations company called Australian American Media. Then in her twenties, she quickly became known as the Australian promoting Australia in the United States. She secured some big clients, such as the America's Cup defence and Australian Tourism, and launched Australian icons like Foster's lager.

It was a good idea and it actually worked. I was in my twenties and like everybody else then I was in there and letting it rip. It was the 1980s. I was really enjoying it and just living for the moment and making the most of every opportunity that came along. Looking back it was an outrageous decision to go and live and work in Los Angeles, but it worked for me.

In Los Angeles with Claudia was her first husband, Richard Keech, who had been her childhood sweetheart. Both of them were consumed by work and there was little time to think of much else apart from the next PR campaign. As Claudia said, she had not ruled out children – she was just too busy to think about them. Also, she thought that she could wait into her thirties because, physically, she had been a late developer. Now in her forties, her skin clear and her hair pulled into two playful plaits, she looks at least ten years younger.

You could say that I was a bit of a late bloomer. When everyone else was having their first teenage date I looked like their little sister. So I didn't do too well in the beginning in that way. I can remember all the girls saying you should wear a bra but I didn't have anything to put in one. I was quite sporty but physically I was tiny. So I wasn't aware of getting old because you react to what you see in the mirror. I have never really felt old or ageing. Also, I didn't know whether I could have a child because I had grown so late. I hadn't tried to have one and I hadn't tried not to have one. Anyway, I was having a great life and like a lot of women today that is the way life is — whether you want a child or not, you don't know whether you can have one until you try.

But it wasn't a child that was to initially interrupt her busy working life. In the late 1980s, Claudia was diagnosed with chronic fatigue syndrome. The usually indefatigable PR whiz was stopped in her tracks. Work faded into the background as Claudia struggled to shake off the extreme tiredness that forced her to bed. She couldn't even make it to the letterbox, let alone think about work. At one point she had to take her own oxygen onto aeroplanes when she flew. She stopped menstruating and her weight fell to 45 kilos.

It was debilitating in the extreme for someone like me who is very motivated. You just can't get your head around it because your head is quite capable of saying, I am going to do this — but your body just isn't listening.

Claudia was forced to take four years off work to rest. She started using both modern and alternative medicine to help build up her immune system, and eventually her customary health and vigour returned.

Sadly, her illness, the intensity of life in Los Angeles, and her husband's own health problems had taken a toll on their marriage. The relationship broke down and Claudia returned to Australia in the early 1990s. She met a new partner, Roger, and within six months of starting their relationship, she was pregnant. 'I got a pleasant surprise,' says Claudia, who by then was in her late thirties.

But Claudia's happiness was short-lived. Thirteen weeks into the pregnancy, she miscarried. The miscarriage was the result of a blighted ovum, which occurs when the placenta and amniotic sac develop and send out pregnancy hormones but the foetus itself does not grow.

For any woman who has had a miscarriage, it is devastating. I was in the hospital having an ultrasound when I found out. My body still felt pregnant; I had swollen breasts.

I had physically gone into pregnancy mode so from that moment my maternal switch was on. Up until then I did not really say I wanted to get pregnant, it was more a case of I would love to have a baby sometime.

I was working when it happened and very few people know about it. It strengthened my relationship with Roger very fast and made two people realise they wanted to be parents and be together. I was living in Mosman in Sydney and there were lots of people with babies. I was so tuned into babies and looking a little bit longingly because now I knew that maybe I could not have a successful pregnancy. But the button a lot of people might feel a lot earlier was not only on for me, it was flashing like a neon sign!

Claudia and Roger decided to get married. They both believed they wanted to have children together and started trying to conceive.

I got pregnant instantly. I believe it was meant to be. Roger was meant to be the father of Callan – that sounds a little bit cosmic but that is how I felt about it. Just because of the way I fell pregnant and how quickly it happened.

Then in her early forties, Claudia, fit and healthy, had a trouble-free pregnancy. She says the medical fraternity treated her well, despite her being in the 'at risk' age group of 35 plus. Like many older mothers, Claudia bridles at being called an elderly primiparae (that is, a woman who is giving birth for the first time). Actually, the term made Claudia laugh – it seemed rather archaic and not at all connected to the way she felt about herself.

When you hear the name that describes older mothers you feel as if you should get out your walking frame. It's weird because I really didn't feel old and I certainly didn't look it. I used to joke with my obstetrician, and ask him if he knew any other geri- atric mums I could hang out with. At the end of my pregnancy, he told me that in the time that I had been seeing him, half his practice was women over 35. So I certainly wasn't the odd one out.

As an older mother-to-be, Claudia knew it would be prudent to have screening or diagnostic tests to check the health of the foetus. But after her miscarriage she was concerned about the risks involved. Both diagnostic tests – chorionic villus sampling and amniocentesis – carry a small risk of miscarriage, with the risk associated with CVS slightly higher. Claudia decided she would not have a CVS but agreed to an amniocentesis at 20 weeks. She had also considered an elective Caesarean because of her age, but ultimately decided to attempt a natural birth. However, after 21 hours of labour, her cervix only 2 centimetres dilated and her baby showing the first signs of stress, Claudia had an emergency Caesarean. Callan was born on 24 June 1995.

The arrival of her hard-won late baby was a time of great joy for Claudia. Almost nine years later her mind is still clear on how she feels about having Callan in her life.

I can categorically say it is the best thing I have ever done in my life. My career really looked after me, it was great. But the best thing I have ever done in my life? Having this child, definitely. As an older mum I am absolutely sure of that.

Now in her late forties, Claudia is considering reducing her working week so she can spend more time with Callan, go to his school concerts and sports days and share his favourite hobbies such as boogie boarding. But Claudia has had to steer around quite a few obstacles to reach this point and she agrees that, in some ways, being older has given her the wisdom to know which way to step and when.

For example, she says being older helped her manage life as a single mother. Not long after Callan was born she and Roger divorced. He now has infrequent contact with Callan. Claudia remained a single mum for three years until she met and married her third husband, Michael Harris.

Being older, she says, also helped her recognise when the job–family juggle just wasn't working. She recalls how busy her working life was back then – for example, she flew to America to organise a Hollywood film premiere when Callan was just under a year old. He went with her and she hired a nanny to look after him during the day while she worked. In Sydney she was working from her home office so she could breastfeed, but she still had to attend meetings and call on clients.

I didn't feel the pressure to work and be a mother from anyone else – I put it on myself. I also needed an income as a single mum. I was working hard and doing things with Callan that were important to me as a mum. But at one point I became aware of just what other modern mums are going through and that's why I started motherInc. I noticed that Callan was doing okay, the job was doing okay, but I wasn't doing so well. I was getting run-down.

Somewhere along the line I had not made the transition to full-time working mum as successfully as one could. But I don't really know if anyone can do that without some kind of support system, and I don't know if age makes that much of a difference.

What I have learned from motherInc is that parents generally and mothers especially have to prepare themselves for a major change when they have children. There is no warning. The more people you talk to who are mothers the better, because you just don't know how you will handle it. You don't know if you will be able to pop back to work three or six months later. You don't know what little genetic blueprint you are going to get.

When Callan was almost three, Claudia knew her life wasn't

working for her. She loved being a mum, but she didn't like the fact that there was simply no time for her own life outside work and family commitments. The juggle had become more difficult as Callan got older – as Claudia and other mothers know well, babies tend to be less of a challenge than toddlers as they spend a lot of time sleeping and are relatively immobile.

When they are babies you have a routine and if you have a babysitter you know they are sleeping a lot and you learn to manage their health and yours. But when they become toddlers there is much more interaction, it creeps up on you and you need to do more with them. Plus you are trying to stop them suiciding every ten seconds – you can't stop watching them for a second.

Callan was in child care three days a week and there was not an ounce of guilt putting him there because he loved it. So he was fine and work was fine, but I still found whatever was required of me at work during my four-day week creeping into my time with Callan. I was working late at night when Callan was asleep and he had back-to-back ear infections which meant he was waking every four hours or so at night.

During most of this time, Claudia was a single mother. She says this wasn't problematic for her because she could organise her own life and time as she wanted. Her world revolved around Callan and her permanent part-time work at Murdoch Magazines, where she'd been since Callan was 20 months old. There, she helped launch *Men's Health* and created public relations strategies for *New Woman* and *marie claire*.

The crunch came when Claudia started a relationship with Michael.

What tipped me over was meeting the man who was going to be my husband. We started having a full social life, which a lot of parents do. But I hadn't had that before. When I didn't have another adult to think about I had it sorted. It is like an older woman who has a relationship with a spouse and then a child arrives – everything needs rejigging.

Everything was going well – Callan, the job, the new relationship with Michael. However, Claudia remembers thinking one day, 'There isn't five seconds in my life for me.'

So I took six months off work and in that time I saw every other mother was like me. They only had five seconds for themselves and it was as if no one had caught up with the modern mum. The modern mum has all sorts of pressures now. She could be a woman who is working, and if she isn't, and her husband is, he might be working harder to bring in more income. She gets quite isolated. If she is working she has a mighty juggle on her hands. If she is an older mum there may not be relatives nearby or alive to help out. If they are on a single income, then they can't afford much help.

Claudia used her time off well, and her research showed there was a glaring hole in the market for a website and support service for modern mums that provided information on issues and products. She decided to step out of the corporate world, and with the enthusiasm and support of fifteen other women launched motherInc in May 2001. It was a hectic time. Only a month earlier, in April, she had married Michael.

For many mothers, figuring out how to cope with the

demands of work and family can be the most stressful element in their lives. Claudia was able to ease these pressures on her life by starting motherInc. However, the commitment and assistance of Michael was vital at this time. A partner in a training consultancy business, he opted to reduce his workload so he could be more flexible with his time for the first six months of Claudia's new project.

'Neither of us wanted to employ someone to look after Callan,' he told the *Sunday Telegraph* in December 2001. 'There needed to be a little bit of give, and one of us was going to have to take a step back work-wise.'[1]

Claudia says that being older enabled both her and Michael to look at the situation and make parenting and career choices which satisfied them both. She says she used this mature wisdom again when deciding to merge motherInc.

For mothers like me, whether I was younger or older, I was still going to have a juggle, but because I was older and I had certain skills, I saw what was needed and I did something about it. In this respect, if I was a younger mum I don't think I would have had the professional knowledge to act on. I would have done what a lot of other parents would have done and still do and that's just get on with it. I really think that older mums are more at peace and more confident with the decisions they make.

I also married someone who is in his forties and has seen the world and is one of those people who is naturally good with children. It is not like you plan this sort of thing, but I suppose there was a silent interview going on when I was dating Michael to see if he was good enough to be Callan's stepdad.

Since starting motherInc, Claudia has been outspoken on issues such as child care, parent-friendly workplaces and the need for greater access to maternity leave. She believes strongly that government policy and workplace practice both need to catch up on these issues if there is to be any hope of alleviating the much-discussed 'fertility crisis' in Australia.

In August 2002, Claudia was interviewed about a British poll which found that older mothers were in a state of despair as a result of sleep deprivation, leaving them unable to cope with the demands of work, children and partners. Claudia didn't even bother to feign surprise and turned the blame to government policy – or the lack of it. 'Up until now,' she told the reporter, 'the government's policy has been geared to *The Brady Bunch* and that family model is simply not an accurate reflection of Australian society.'[2] She maintains that governments need to take a closer look at the needs of modern mums.

The thing is, I am different and so is everyone else. You used to have a traditional family where when dad got home he would kiss the kids on the cheek before they went to bed and mum was the managing director of the house. Everyone is different now. I am just one of those women who is different. Most women go to school to have some sort of job or career, not necessarily to smash a glass ceiling. I am just one of those women who left school and got on with achieving. I think it is a juggle now because the majority of women in Australia are choosing to go back to work when children are quite young, and the majority are choosing to be part-time. But it is still a juggle and the reason is mothers today are writing the book on this – there are no rules, whatever your age.

We have to educate the government to come in with the right support services that women and men need. We have to educate our families not to be judgmental because we are doing it differently. We even have to talk to husbands or partners about the fact that mothers may be working part-time while the kids are still young, but they can't actually still do all the housework they used to do when they were home full-time with a baby.

Claudia firmly believes that politicians need to take notice of the major social changes affecting women, in particular their yearning to find some middle ground between career, children and marriage. They ignore the messages that are coming from the electorate regarding family-friendly workplaces and child-care support at their peril.

There is another issue that Claudia believes should not be ignored, and this is the relationship between couples after a child is born. Judging by feedback from women who access motherInc, there is a great deal of anxiety about relationships between spouses after a child is born. A survey in 2003 by Relationships Australia confirmed that dual careers combined with children were putting a huge strain on relationships. Ninety per cent of those surveyed said that the trend towards dual careers was putting relationships in jeopardy because people were not prepared to compromise their individual goals for their relationship or family. Forty per cent of respondents to the survey said that they felt they had no real power to balance work and family.[3] This is an issue that can't be solved by legislation, although it could be alleviated by more flexible working hours for both men and women.

Happily for older parents, Claudia believes they might be

more capable of both identifying the stresses on a relationship and having the experience to take action. Certainly, this has been the case for her and Michael, who have worked hard at keeping their marriage strong.

I worry about modern relationships. We are so good at planning our kids' health and their education when they are little and deciding which crèche they are going to go to and which hobby, but I am not sure we are putting enough into the adult relationship in the house. I think as an older parent I recognise this – if you don't put the hard yards into your relationship with your spouse, your relationship could be in trouble. The demands of children can erode an adult relationship quite dramatically and before you know it you end up with two strangers living in the house.

I don't know if younger people have this privilege of insight, but I will say as an older parent that Michael and I put aside one night a week to go to a movie or have a walk. We need to do this together, to have this shared activity. We have an awareness about our relationship. I am not sure if people in their twenties have those skills on board – you need to know that a relationship will not glide along while all the demands of children impact on it. It will collapse and burn if you don't invest time in it – and that's a guarantee.

Having experienced, albeit late in life, the joys and the frustrations of motherhood, Claudia says she would love to have a second child. Now nearly 50, she fears, however, that she has finally run out of time.

Two years after meeting Michael she checked her options

with an IVF clinic in Sydney, feeling that she may need help to conceive if they decided to have a child together. Despite comments on her youthful appearance, the medical fraternity was discouraging due to her mature age. Claudia was then in her late forties. Even so, she had some tests which showed she was still ovulating and that another pregnancy was not out of the question.

However, the IVF specialist refused to go ahead due to her age and recommended that Claudia try to fall pregnant naturally. He suggested that she speak to a fertility specialist who might be able to suggest other ways for her to improve her fertility. So Claudia contacted a fertility specialist, but her hopes of help were quickly dashed. She says he told her in 'no uncertain terms' over the telephone to 'listen – you are on a fast track to menopause and it isn't going to happen'.

Claudia and Michael had spoken to this same specialist soon after meeting each other, to check their options regarding fertility. He had been equally dismissive at that time, when Claudia was 46.

> I had hoped that medical tests proving I was still ovulating, the obvious fact that my body continued to operate at a youthful level and the referral by my long-term GP and the IVF specialist would mean that my situation may be worth considering by this specialist.
>
> I was appalled at his response and lack of tact in delivering his message – over the telephone – a call made by him, after I had made a simple call to book an appointment with his nurse to come in for a consultation.
>
> At motherInc, the staff, who knew I was checking my options

regarding fertility, were in uproar. One mother who had succeeded in having a child as an older mum on her tenth IVF attempt in the United States confirmed her doctor would have me in the hospital to begin the procedure immediately, given the results of my tests at that time.

I realised that to pursue a possible second pregnancy I would need to leave Australia and to try my chances in the United States. When thinking and talking about this with Michael we both believed that what had begun as an exploration of options had ended as a truly unpleasant experience with the medical world as a result of their treatment of more mature parents.

I have been aware my whole life that my body was operating at a more youthful level than my chronological years. Yet, no one was prepared to take a risk on me, even though Michael and I were ready to give it a go. At this point, with the knowledge that we were both already blessed with the most wonderful son we could ever ask for, we felt relocating our lives to go through IVF in the US was a bridge too far.

I often say if there was a mixing pot to create a child and you were able to pick ingredients or genes you would like to put into the mixing pot, then Callan has all those ingredients. We are blessed to have him in our lives and there really is no need for another baby.

However, for other mature women, who do not have a Callan, I would say don't be put off by the medical world. Pursue your options and dreams wherever they may be – there are mothers having their first child at 46 or 48. While every educated woman knows that at this age you are battling against the odds, it doesn't mean you can't give it a try.

Amanda Ellis

economist and author

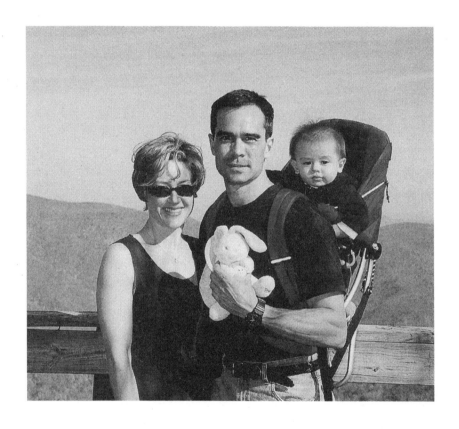

'I think, for me, this has been the best possible time to have a child.'

SINCE AMANDA ELLIS was a child, the business of numbers has figured largely in her life. Her accountant father impressed on her the importance of saving from a young age, and she is a respected economist who has worked in Australia and Europe. Amanda now holds a senior position with the World Bank in Washington, DC. So it's fairly safe to say that she belongs to the no-nonsense world of statistics and balance sheets.

However, when Amanda reflects on the circumstances that led to her becoming a mother at the age of 40, to son Mitchell, this world starts to blur and another picture emerges where fate, coincidence or serendipity – call it what you like – has the upper hand.

If you had to choose someone to personify the ideal of a high-powered businesswoman, then Amanda Ellis would be a perfect fit. In the 1980s she left her native New Zealand to join the diplomatic world, working as a specialist in international trade and development economics at the Organization for Economic Co-operation and Development (OECD) in Paris and the United Nations in Geneva. For ten years she managed international aid programs for women in Vietnam, Laos and Cambodia, before turning her boundless energy and expertise to the business of banking as head of women's markets and national manager for women in business at Westpac Banking Corporation in Sydney.

Added to Amanda's Westpac responsibilities were not only her work for major women's organisations such as the National Breast Cancer Network and the Global Banking Alliance for Women, but also her new role as author. In 2002, Amanda's book, *Women's Business, Women's Wealth*, which focused on her lifelong passion – women creating a life of their own through business and work – became a bestseller.

As part of her work at Westpac, Amanda was required to attend numerous international finance and business conferences and courses. In May 2002, she attended one such course at the Harvard Business School in Boston. It was titled 'Women Leading Business', and top businesswomen from around the world gathered to learn and share their experiences. There were many inspiring speakers, but a speech by one woman in particular was to have a profound effect on Amanda.

One of the women who got up to talk to us was the European head of a large software company. It was a dinner and we all had to share something about ourselves that was personal. She started to talk, then she just burst into tears – which is not the sort of thing you do at the Harvard Business School. Everybody looked at each other.

She said she felt that she had been conned by the corporate world. Everyone just looked at each other again. She then said that she had focused so much of her life on her career that she had no idea she couldn't get the career thing happening, make all the money she wanted and then have a family. She said she was 44 and nobody had told her about declining fertility, which I know sounds kind of wild. But as she said to us, it is not something that you think about. She was very emotional about the whole subject.

I was 39 at the time and I just thought having children wasn't at the top of my agenda. I wasn't with the right person when I was in my thirties and I just thought that it wasn't meant to be.

Later at the dinner this same woman came up to speak to me and one of the other younger women. She said to me, 'I just want you to know that not making a decision [about having children] is making a decision.'

At the time I didn't really care one way or another if I had children or not. I was so focused on my career. I said to her that was how I felt and she just said to me, 'That was how I felt at your age, too, and now I really regret not having children. Think about that while you still have a choice.'

Almost two years later, Amanda considers that Harvard encounter to have been a catalyst for change in her life.

She planted this seed in my mind. Before then I had also interviewed veterinary surgeon Dr Judith Slocombe, Telstra Businesswoman of the Year for 2001/2002 – and a mother of nine children – and we had talked about this very subject of career and children. She said to me that there was no right time to have children, that you can't plan for every eventuality.

A few days after the Harvard course Amanda happened to pick up a copy of *Time* magazine. It included an article about the very issue which had been at the heart of the woman's emotional outburst over dinner – the potentially disastrous effect of declining fertility on a career-focused woman's hopes of having a family in her late thirties or early forties.

The magazine story had been inspired by a book by economist Sylvia Ann Hewlett called *Creating a Life: Professional Women and the Quest for Children* (published in Australia as *Baby Hunger*). The book had sparked an emotional debate among feminists and conservatives in the United States and Great Britain. Were the women who had postponed having children in favour of a career really in danger of emotional peril because of age-related infertility? Or was this just another conservative plot to stifle women's rights to equal choice? Either way, the book severely dented the myth that women had it all and that the increasing incidence of childlessness in countries such as Australia, Britain and the United States was voluntary. The *Time* story tracked the debate and illustrated the pincer-like effect on a generation of women resulting from the trend to delay childbirth, for whatever reason, and the natural depletion of fertility as women aged.

Amanda read the story and, having a head for figures, took particular note of the statistics relating to women her age or slightly older. The story told her that once a woman celebrated her forty-second birthday, the chances of her having a baby with her own eggs, even with advanced medical help, were less than

10 per cent. By age 40, half of her eggs are chromosomally abnormal, and by 42 that figure rises to 90 per cent, meaning a very high risk of miscarriage.[1]

> *I realised that there was a small chance of me being able to conceive naturally because I was almost 40 at the time. I thought, oh well, that's fine, I don't need to use contraception any more. So I went off the contraceptive pill.*

At the time, Amanda was living in Australia and her husband, Keric Blaine, a lawyer with the American Air Force, was living in the United States. They had only been married for two years, but had known each other since their mid-twenties, becoming engaged in 1988 after meeting at graduate school in Hawaii. Amanda says they knew then that they were soul mates, but earthly distractions got in the way of their romance.

> *I didn't want to be an air force wife and I then went into foreign affairs and Keric didn't want to be a diplomatic husband. We commuted between countries for three years then he married someone else and had children. I went off to work at the OECD in Paris. We met again in 2000 and this time we decided to get married and work out where to live later.*

In June, a month after the Harvard course, they met briefly in Hawaii, before Amanda went back to Australia.

> *I had just gone off the pill but it was the wrong time in my cycle for anything to happen anyway so I didn't think anything of it. I went off to speak at a conference in Malaysia and then back*

to Australia where I was getting ready to do media for the launch of my book, Women's Business, Women's Wealth. *It was weird, but I woke up a couple of times during that week when I got to Australia with this really strange feeling in my stomach. I thought it must be butterflies about the book.*

The first interview I did for television was on regional TV in Newcastle and the moment I walked into the studio the hair and make-up guy said, 'Hello darl, where's your baby?' I said, 'I beg your pardon?' He said: 'Haven't you just had a baby?' I sucked in my stomach and said I was sorry, but I didn't know what he meant. I thought I was looking pretty taut, trim and terrific. He said, 'If you haven't just had a baby you must be pregnant – you have a baby in your aura.' I said, 'I have a baby in my what?' I told him I was an economist and I didn't buy that sort of stuff. Then I started spouting all these statistics about how I couldn't get pregnant at my age. He said to me, 'You can spout all the statistics you like but I have a gift for this and I have been right nine times out of nine in the last two years and you are number ten. And it is a boy so you might as well get on with it.' I think I turned really green right there and then because the media person looked a bit surprised when she saw me and told me I was supposed to be looking better after make-up, not worse!

The next day Amanda decided to do a home pregnancy test. It gave a positive result. She couldn't believe it. Next stop was the doctor to ask how this could have happened.

He said to me that the conception date was 18 June, which was the night I arrived in Hawaii. Abnormally, I was having a

32-day cycle. He said I would not have fallen pregnant under normal circumstances. The whole thing was very freaky and Keric and I decided it was meant to be.

I was a little nonplussed by it all because the circumstances under which I found out were so strange. When I rang my husband he was wonderful and said he thought it was fantastic. He asked me how I felt and I said I wasn't sure. I was uncertain about the whole thing because I just hadn't expected it at all given all those statistics. It was certainly a surprise. It is very disconcerting for an economist when you fall outside the standard bell curve distribution. From a work point of view it was disruptive, but I look back now and I think with all those weird coincidences — especially the make-up man — it all seems like it was fate writ large. I am a very rational person most of the time but this was one of those times when you have to suspend belief and say I don't have anything to do with this. It was meant to be.

Amanda was 39 when she found out she was pregnant. She had mixed feelings about this unexpected development. Not one to renege on any work obligations, she was worried that she would not be able to meet the publicity commitments for her book. Also, a part of her was a little apprehensive about motherhood. After all, although she had many good friends who were mothers, she had hardly thought of herself in that role. Her focus had been on helping women develop businesses and pursue careers. She knew from her own experience that the very time in a woman's life when, physically, it is right for her to have a child, is also the time she needs to focus on her career. That focus had been made stronger in Amanda by her lifelong passion for helping women improve their economic situation. She recalls how the seed for this passion had been planted during her years at a private girls school in Dunedin, New Zealand. It was a good school academically, but the headmistress had a very old-fashioned idea of what a 'young lady' needed to learn to get on in life.

We had classes on bathing babies and painting our fingernails. It was all about accomplishments a young lady needed to get married, and it really annoyed me. From that time on I realised it was important to be an individual. My parents encouraged me in this way too. My mother, Natalie, worked when it was frowned upon. She had wanted to be a lawyer but her father had told her that girls could only be teachers, nurses or secretaries. She became a teacher. She instilled in me the belief that women of my generation had the opportunity to create their own lives and the opportunity to be financially independent as well and that they could call the shots.

Encouraged by her parents, Amanda set out to achieve financial independence, and to advise other women how to achieve it too. By the time she reached her late thirties she had all the accroutrements of corporate success, including the maximum annual bonus for her performance at Westpac for achieving 200 per cent of targets. Amanda gave her undivided attention to her career, which, combined with the fact that she hadn't met the right man, meant that having children was not on the agenda.

I wasn't with the right person through my thirties and I thought if it wasn't meant to be for me to have children, then it wasn't meant to be. I had come from a small family [she is an only child] and I didn't have any maternal urges. I had thought about adopting as something I could do at a later age if I felt that I really wanted to have a child. I sponsored a number of refugees and children who had lost their parents in landmine accidents. I had thought it would be wonderful to make the life of just one of these children better, so this had been on my mind since about 1996 when I first went to Cambodia.

Amanda recalls her conversation with Dr Judith Slocombe and how they had talked about careers and kids and how pointless it was to apply any kind of timing to becoming a mother. Dr Slocombe spoke of how she had juggled starting a new business, working 16 hours a day, and looking after her large family.

I told her that career had been my priority and I was probably a bit old to have children. She repeated to me that there was never a right time to do this. She said to make a list of the five most important things in life and if having a child was in that top five then get on and do it.

I asked Amanda if, back then, she felt just like the kind of woman Sylvia Ann Hewlett had written about in her book – the highly successful businesswoman who had it all except children. 'Yes,' she said. 'When I read the article on her book I thought, "Oh my God, that is just like me."'

Even though Amanda recognised herself in Hewlett's book, her reaction was not to rush out and get pregnant. She took the philosophical approach, tossed her contraceptive pills and decided what will be will be.

Also, Keric had two children from his previous marriage and he hadn't shown any desire for more. For these reasons Amanda had decided against fertility treatments like IVF. She had also seen a number of girlfriends experience IVF: the injections, the waiting and the disappointment, and decided it was not for her.

I just thought that wasn't something I wanted to go through and I didn't feel strongly enough about having my own biological child.

However, Amanda says she was caught by surprise when she read the *Time* story about age-related infertility.

I wasn't aware of the way fertility drops and how some career women were feeling about this whole issue until the Harvard course. And then I read the article in Time. *I know this sounds naive but I only had a vague idea of what happens to a woman's fertility. I didn't realise the full extent of it.*

Then again, the statistics didn't matter in her case. She fell pregnant against the odds. Even though this shook the rational economist in her, Amanda once again took a philosophical approach and decided it was fate. She continued to work hard during her pregnancy almost to the day that Mitchell was born. She had moved, temporarily, to the United States to have the baby and was working at home on projects for Westpac. Being an older mother she'd had concerns about miscarriage and abnormalities, but she had a healthy pregnancy and was treated well by her doctors in Australia. However this changed when she arrived in the United States.

The first doctor I saw [in the United States] was a young guy who said to me in this drawl, 'Well, ma'am, the good Lord meant women to have babies in their twenties, not your advanced age.' He told me about all the possibilities of all the defects that my baby could have, which terrified me. I could have hit him — I was so angry.

I ended up having a Caesarean. I was scheduled to have the baby at a military hospital — Bethesda Naval Hospital — but two days before my waters broke, all the staff there were sent off to the Persian Gulf for the war in Iraq.

So they couldn't take me and I had to be diverted to another army hospital which was not a maternity hospital. I had a 27-hour labour and then a Caesarean so the birth wasn't such a fantastic experience.

In the US you're out very fast — two days after a C-section — and you don't get to see a doctor again for another six weeks. There is no follow-up support at home, either, so it was a huge shock dealing with my milk coming in, breastfeeding, etc. A couple of wonderful women who had children a few months older came to my rescue and I shall be eternally grateful.

When Amanda fell pregnant she realised that her life was going to change — she knew little about babies but enough to know that life, as she knew it, was never going to be the same. She wasn't to realise how great the change would be.

Career has always been important to Amanda, and even though she loved being a mum to Mitchell she didn't want to let that part of her life go. She knew she was not a stay-at-home mum. She fully intended to keep up the pace of work at Westpac after she returned from maternity leave, and in August

2003, six months after Mitchell was born, Amanda was back in Australia running a financial conference for Westpac. Keric came to the conference to babysit.

It was a women in leadership conference and everyone decided that Mitchell was the conference baby. I don't know if it would have been the same environment if it had been a male-dominated conference.

Despite her hard work and commitment during her years at Westpac and her desire to stay with the organisation, as she wanted her husband and child to eventually live in Australia, Amanda left the bank in late 2003. She cannot talk in detail about the circumstances of her departure, which followed a management restructure by a new boss when she was on leave after Mitchell was born. However, she says her experience confirmed to her the vital need for every woman at every level in a company to know her rights in the workplace.

It is really disconcerting in Australia as there appear to be more and more instances of discrimination against women who have children. It is the kind of thing that you think will never happen to me. But it can and it does. A new boss when you're physically out of the workplace and anything can happen. All you have to do is read books like Anne Summers's The End of Equality *to realise there is a real danger that we are going backwards in Australia.*

It is important to protect the rights that Australian women do have in the workplace and I believe it is a shame that Australia doesn't have a universal maternity benefit, although some companies opt to pay it on a voluntary basis. [At the time of writing, Australia and the United States are the only two OECD countries that don't have a national paid maternity scheme.]

However every woman has the right to return to the same job she had before she went on leave after having a child. That is the law. We need to protect those rights. It is vital to know what the Australian law is in regard to this and also to touch base with your union representative before you go on leave so you have someone who you can contact if a problem arises. I had never been a big fan of unions but after my experience at Westpac I changed my mind.

The union [Financial Sector Union of Australia – FSU] contacted me when I went on maternity leave and said we just want to stay in touch to make sure if there are any anomalies then we are there to help. I never expected to need to take them up on the offer, but boy, was I glad I had the FSU to turn to when both I and one of my former staff, who had had twins, experienced the same thing at work after having a baby.

The FSU was great about providing free legal advice and pointing out that it was important for individual women to ensure their legal rights were upheld on behalf of all women. It just helps to know that you have somebody bigger than you to fight on your behalf if necessary, and situating it in the context of a wider struggle certainly helps give you perspective.

It is perhaps ironic that Amanda, who has spent her life working to give women independence and strength in the workplace, felt powerless against certain changes that happened at Westpac which effectively led her to leave a job that she loved. In retrospect she learned a valuable management lesson that she says should be emphasised to the upper echelons of business.

> *If you treat women well on maternity leave I think you probably have incredible loyalty for life. On the other hand, if you have a bad experience then you can feel disillusioned.*

Amanda says that as a new mum, she was on something of an emotional rollercoaster at the time, fuelled by sleep deprivation, making it all the more difficult to deal with what was happening at Westpac. To make matters worse, she was in the United States, and Westpac management was in Australia. She felt bolstered, however, by her friends and her own sense of self-worth.

> *Being older was absolutely an advantage for me at this point. If I had been younger and less bolshie I would have thought, 'Oh my goodness it must be me or something that I have done.' I think being older you recognise that this kind of thing is systemic, and of course I had the evidence of the maximum bonus for my performance to remind myself it was not performance-related. I also had a lot of close girlfriends who were a wonderful support network. That was one of the advantages of having a child later in life – I could draw on their advice and knowledge.*

Being older also meant Amanda had the philosophical strength to deal with what happened to her. Just as importantly, it meant she had the expertise to find another job. Her role at the World Bank is to advance private sector development and gender issues within the bank and its investment arm, the International Finance Corporation. This chance to champion women's entrepreneurship worldwide is a dream job for Amanda, who has taken to the task with typical energy and enthusiasm. She attended her first international conference with the World Bank in December 2003 in Nigeria, then went on to Jordan to help train Iraqi women leaders, including the two women members of the interim Governing Council.

Of course, Mitchell went with her. Having spent the first six months at home with him, working on projects for Westpac, Amanda is now working full-time in Washington, DC. Each day sounds like a mini marathon.

We get up at 5.30 am (ugh!) to be able to leave the house by 6.30 am, drop Mitchell at daycare by 7 am so we are able to get to the metro and in to work by around 7.45 am. My husband and I try to coordinate leaving work at the same time so we can pick Mitchell up together and have some time to talk on the way home – once we're home we take turns cooking dinner or bathing him so we can get him into bed by 7.30 pm. We have been worried that despite two naps the days are very long for a one year old, so we recently arranged with the 18-year-old daughter of our daycare provider to take Mitchell home around 4.30, bath him and give him dinner so we can have more quality time with him when we get home. This seems to be working pretty well so far.

I guess nothing could have prepared me for the incredible fatigue of baby and work, especially when a few nocturnal teething episodes coincide with an important meeting or presentation! That's when I'm really grateful for close friends' advice that this is the hardest time and that you start to 'come out of the tiredness tunnel' around the one year mark. That has certainly been true for us. We've got better at outsourcing, too, realising that we just cannot manage to do everything ourselves and stay sane! So now we pay a cleaner to come in once a week and we have that regular afternoon care as well as full-time day care. It's expensive, but the peace of mind is worth it.

Moving to the US just prior to Mitchell's birth meant coming to terms with a whole new system (I appreciate Australia's medical system even more now!), making new friends and also establishing myself in a new job. The toughest thing was not having my support network of wonderful friends, many of whom had recently had babies and were a wealth of good advice and much needed tips. When I started my new role, I had presumed I would be able to put Mitchell in day care at the World Bank, but there is a very long waiting list – we were number 405 to be precise! We actually found our home day care provider through our real estate agent, whose granddaughter attended and really enjoyed it.

Mitchell absolutely loves day care, and he's a very social little boy who enjoys the other children. It's very much a family atmosphere. I feel Mitchell is getting so much more out of this experience than I could have offered as an inexperienced and isolated new mother in new surroundings.

We thought it would be better for me to go back to work sooner rather than later and it was a fantastic job opportunity as it is hard to get into the World Bank. I am loving it. I don't feel like superwoman – I just feel exhausted. I call it a grinding fatigue. A girlfriend said to me that sleep deprivation is like being drunk – everyone else notices it except you.

Amanda also felt the need to return to a working environment which has been part of her life for two decades. These habits are hard to break, even if you are faced with the prospect of mind-numbing fatigue due to loss of sleep and teething babies.

Financially I needed to go back to work and I also wanted to go back to work for myself. I am not a stay-at-home person and I feel that Mitchell gets a lot of stimulation at day care that I can't provide.

Amanda says she relies heavily on Keric to share the care of Mitchell. She says he has been crucial in enabling her to be a mother and to work in a demanding job located in an inter-national hub like Washington DC.

My husband Keric is absolutely amazing with Mitchell, and we both feel we share parenting duties pretty evenly. On weekends we tend to spend most of our time with other friends who have little ones, too. It's inevitable that you gravitate towards others with small children. Mitchell is incredibly active (or is it just that I am getting old and slow!) and started careening around like a little drunken sailor at about 11 months, clapping his hands delightedly at his newfound mobility. We have a playroom set up for him with kiddie gates, but he much prefers 'escaping' and wreaking havoc in the rest of the house, drawn like a magnet to things like plugs and cords. It has been a real process of trial and error, but I think we're pretty much kiddie-proof now.

Between her job at the World Bank and being a mum to Mitchell, Amanda has little time in her life at the moment to think about much else. But she has contemplated the question which seems to hover around all first-time mothers, particularly those who have left having a child until later in life: should she have a second baby?

The economist in Amanda has done the figures, looking at the fact that she and Keric have a mortgage and he must continue to financially support his two other children from an earlier marriage. Plus she has a new and demanding job. The rational decision was to stay with one child.

> *I really wanted to have a second child after Mitchell was born but we weighed it up financially and we had to ask ourselves: were we able to do this, as well as our other commitments, and give these children everything we wanted to give them? I am not sure about that. Also, I guess it was one of those things that we needed to do really fast. I am now 41 and if it was going to happen again it might not happen as quickly as it did the first time.*

Despite the fact that she feels she has left it too late to have another child, Amanda has no regrets about having her first baby at 40. She says being older has helped her cope in many ways, especially with the work–family juggle and knowing what was best for her and her child, rather than paying attention to what others thought she should do.

> *If I'd had a child earlier I don't know if I would have known how to juggle everything. I think I also had a lot to prove in a career sense and I wouldn't have felt comfortable having to juggle those two things back then. Now I feel very comfortable that*

I know I can continue my work and my life purpose to help empower women financially. That is what really drives me. Now I have an opportunity to do that and I am blessed to have a family life as well that three or four years ago I almost missed out on. I think, for me, this has been the best possible time to have a child.

Amanda wants all women – especially new mothers – to be financially independent. For her expert financial advice on how to get the best out of your workplace and superannuation, see page 307.

Deborah Claxton

celebrity agent

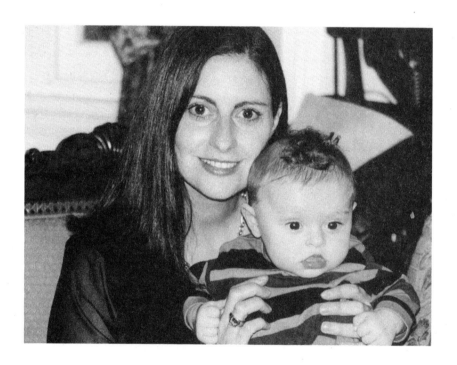

‘Having IVF was something I had to do . . .
I had an overwhelming desire to have a child
and have a family and I believed in my heart
that it would happen. It was never on my
mind to stop.’

DEBORAH CLAXTON can remember when she was told she was pregnant in early 2001. She was 39 and desperately wanted a baby. At last it seemed as if her hopes were to be realised.

However, she had reason to be cautious – Deborah had been pregnant twice before, once after having conceived naturally and another time after in-vitro fertilisation. On both occasions she lost her baby.

Determined to become a mother, she had continued with IVF despite miscarrying. It was on her fifth IVF treatment that Deborah fell pregnant again. Her past history was a concern, but Deborah felt intuitively that this time her pregnancy would be successful and she would finally become a mother.

From the moment that I was told I was pregnant I knew that

I would be fine. It was just a feeling that I had – this time everything would be okay.

Call it women's intuition, but Deborah was right. On 12 November 2001, she gave birth to her son, Will, who weighed a healthy 2.9 kilos. Beside her in the maternity ward of a Sydney hospital was her husband, Phill McMartin. It had been a smooth birth but there was one small hiccup – Will had arrived almost three weeks early meaning Deborah didn't have a break between managing her Sydney-based business and becoming a mum. She didn't mind. After four years of trying to have a child, at one time contemplating adoption, Deborah was simply grateful that Will had been born.

Will is now two years old and Deborah is working four days a week managing Claxton Speakers Bureau. Her company secures professional speaking engagements for the eminent men and women it represents, including business and political leaders, media and sporting personalities and authors, as well as motivational speakers. Dr Jose Ramos Horta, the Nobel Peace Prize winner and East Timor's Foreign Minister, journalists Maxine McKew and Sally Loane, scientist Dr Karl Kruszelnicki, Justice Marcus Einfeld and former Children's Court Magistrate Barbara Holborow are just a few of the dynamos on her books.

It's a busy and thriving business, and a highlight of 2003 was being appointed as the supplier of speakers and entertainment for the official corporate hospitality events for the Rugby World Cup.

Deborah is proud of its success, having set up the business in 1996 after managing celebrity agent Harry M. Miller's speakers bureau. Her husband, Phill, works in the business with her, having joined forces with his wife just before Will was born.

It's a hectic life and the fact that she has her own business adds a different set of pressures to Deborah's workaday world. Even so, Deborah always has time for Will, her 'miracle child' who was born largely out of her determination to beat the biological clock. But for a while there it looked as if the biological clock was going to be the victor in this fertility tussle.

Deborah's inability to fall pregnant naturally was due to age-related infertility. Before she had IVF she'd gone through tests which confirmed this was the case. The facts were there in front of her: it looked as if she had left her attempt at having children too late.

True, she was only 36 when she and Phill started to try to conceive, and in her late thirties when she started IVF. For some women this might not have been a problem. But it was for Deborah and she realised only too late that her timing, when it came to motherhood, was way off the mark. She had thought she could wait to be a mother.

Deborah's plan in her mid-thirties was to get her business up and running, get married to Phill, buy a house and then progress to parenthood. Not an unfamiliar strategy for many women in their thirties. Besides, Deborah wasn't previously with the right partner for parenthood, saying part of the reason she left having a baby until later in life was because 'Prince Charming hadn't come along, until Phill'.

I met Phill when I was 30. While both of us wanted to have a committed relationship with marriage and children, we didn't really think that we had to do it all immediately. When you are 30 you don't think about it like that — it seems as if it is a natural progression that all these things will happen eventually.

Also, too, I think it is a generational thing. People look younger, they act younger. I have a lot of girlfriends who are in their mid-forties who look fantastic.

I started my business in 1996 and we got married in the September of that year and it was around the following year that the light went on in my head about having a child. I thought that if I keep going like this we will never stop. We may as well think about having a family and if it happens, it happens — and if it doesn't, it doesn't.

There was no great concern until I fell pregnant and I miscarried.

Deborah had her first miscarriage at about five weeks. I asked her how this affected her. What feelings did it trigger?

Fear. I had never been pregnant before in my life and I started to wonder if there was a reason why this hadn't happened. You start to go through all these different thoughts. I went and spoke to my gynaecologist and he said to give it twelve months and then we will look at this again. I was happy with that advice because having gone through a miscarriage I realised that it can be such a normal thing in pregnancy. Many women experience some kind of difficulty with pregnancy.

True, up to 20 per cent of women will suffer a miscarriage, and 5 per cent will suffer multiple miscarriages. Medical science is yet to pinpoint why certain miscarriages occur, but the cause can be a genetic abnormality in the foetus. The risk of miscarriage increases with a woman's age so that a 40-year-old woman has a 36 per cent chance of miscarrying.

At 36, Deborah thought she could afford another year of trying to conceive naturally. Twelve months later she was back sitting in front of her gynaecologist.

I started thinking, 'Why isn't this happening?' and a little bit of anxiety crept in. When I went back to my specialist he said he didn't want to waste more time, the reality was that I was now 37 and that my fertility rate was dropping quite dramatically.

Deborah's next step was to visit a fertility specialist, who told her that her chances of conceiving naturally were diminishing. Even with some kind of fertility treatment, such as IVF, the odds were stacked against her falling pregnant and carrying the baby to term.

He sat me down and showed me some statistics and my heart just dropped. He told me that at my age fertility decreases dramatically. He told me that the success rate for fertility treatment was less than 20 per cent for women of my age. Also there was close to a 40 to 50 per cent chance that I could miscarry.

It was difficult to hear this but now I wonder if they tell you to prepare you for IVF because it is something you need to be open-minded about if you are going to do it.

Deborah decided to go ahead with IVF. Before this she had looked at other ways of improving her fertility, such as natural therapies. However she decided it was time to look at the statistics and tests that had been done and face the facts: her chances of conceiving naturally were fairly slim.

If I was in my early thirties, perhaps I would have delayed having IVF because I had more time on my hands, but as each year went past my chances of having a child were diminishing.

Deborah says she wasn't concerned about having IVF, although she was a little surprised to find herself among the growing number of Australian women having fertility treatment: 'I wasn't worried about it — I just thought it would never happen to me.'

Besides, any concerns Deborah may have had about IVF were overshadowed by her need to have a child. She had even applied for adoption papers in case IVF did not work out.

I wouldn't say that the need to have a child became over-whelming, it is just that it shifted on the agenda. When a specialist tells you that you are of a certain age and there is a possibility you won't have a child on your own and you will need assistance, you go looking at all other areas. I can remember at this time there was a little baby girl left in a cardboard box at a hospital somewhere in rural Australia and I said to Phill that if I found that baby I would keep it. He looked at me and said, 'No you wouldn't.' And I said, 'Yes I would.' Because it would have solved all my problems.

Many women who have had IVF, even those who successfully give birth, talk about how the treatment can be emotionally and physically draining. How it can be a marathon journey punctuated by hope and crushing disappointment. And yet it is also irresistible if the need to have a child is great. After all, who can turn their back on hope?

Deborah undertook her IVF treatment with a stoic determination. She wanted a child and she was going to live through what it took to get one. She even managed to look on the bright side.

Having IVF was something I had to do. The disappointment that I experienced was obvious. Having a failed fertility treatment was more painful than I had ever anticipated.

You don't go through any medical procedure thinking it won't work. I just thought it would work. And I always had a positive attitude. I would say to people that I am just trying to have a baby. I don't have a life-threatening illness, it is just for the joy of having a child.

So, right from the beginning I thought I will do whatever it takes to have that child. And I won't give up. If it means I have to keep going then that is what I am going to do.

Deborah maintained this strength of purpose even though her hopes to have a child using IVF were to receive an early setback. After the second cycle of IVF she had a miscarriage. She admits she had initially assumed that IVF would fix everything that was wrong with her fertility.

But it didn't. I was disappointed after this miscarriage but it didn't stop me from going ahead with another cycle of IVF. I had an overwhelming desire to have a child and have a family and

I believed in my heart that it would happen. It was never on my mind to stop.

Yet, considering this miscarriage and her disappointment in not being able to conceive naturally, I had to wonder if she felt as if she had been shortchanged by life. After all, she had done all the right things, hadn't she? She had worked hard at her career to become a successful celebrity agent and had waited until she met the right man for her before she decided to settle down and have children. And yet, here she was facing the very real possibility that she might not have a child.

I felt cheated. I grew up in the country and I was engaged at a young age and thought I would be married and have three children by the time I was 25. All that changed when I moved to Sydney in my early twenties and discovered what an amazing city it is and what an amazing world we live in. I hadn't really thought about this early part of my life and how it could have been so different until this happened to me.

I always felt thrilled for other people when they had children but secretly I had this longing to be a mother and being faced with the reality that there is a problem with your fertility exaggerates the situation in your mind a lot more.

I wouldn't blame anyone specifically for cheating me – just life. I just thought at the time that this sucks.

I wouldn't have changed my life, though. I am a great believer that things happen for a reason. I had never thought about getting married for the sake of getting married or ever having a family with someone whom I didn't adore.

Phill is two years older than Deborah and she says that having children wasn't originally high on his agenda. However, after they married he wanted a family and he supported her decision to have IVF, even if it may have been rough going at times.

> *As a female going through IVF you do tend to forget about your partner and their feelings and you do get a little angry at them and wonder if they understand what is happening to you. My specialist had to point out to me that Phill is a man and I am a woman and we will never think the same. That helped.*

Deborah says that staying busy at work also helped during those years when she was riding the IVF rollercoaster. Being older and having established her own business was an advantage at this time because it gave her the flexibility to take time off to undergo fertility treatment, which included surgery under a general anaesthetic when an egg pick-up had to be performed.

> *I do not think it would have been the same if I worked for a large multinational company. They may be supportive of women who are pregnant, but you still feel as if you have this commitment to someone else. That pressure was alleviated by having my own business and the team who work with me knew what I was going through when I was having IVF. I couldn't have done it without their support.*
>
> *Is this a benefit of being older? In hindsight, while you never plan things, if I hadn't miscarried and instead had that baby when I was 36 my business may not be what it is today. I often*

reflect on that and I think things were meant to happen this way because Phill joined the business which allowed me to step away from it for a short time and work part-time for the first year of Will's life.

Having my own successful business didn't make much of a difference when it came to the financial pressures of IVF. When you have your own business you tend to reinvest back into your business. But I guess we were older and in a secure financial situation. We were both professionals. We had no other major commitments so that our income, apart from our mortgage, was pretty much disposable income. So you choose what to do with that income, whether you want to travel or spend it on renovations.

And there is wonderful government support, too. I was in a situation where I didn't have to pay any money upfront. The IVF clinic would process the rebate and then you pay the balance, which was between $2000 and $3000 for each IVF treatment.

Having IVF is like anything you have to budget for. It was a case of 'When can I do the next one – mentally, emotionally, physically and financially?' When you have two people working towards it, then it is not unobtainable. You just choose not to do other things.

When Deborah finally fell pregnant with Will she felt as if a weight had been lifted from her shoulders. She hadn't realised how all those years of trying to get pregnant, either naturally or with IVF, had taken a toll on her. She had gained weight and despite the success of her business there was emptiness in her life. Almost three years later she remembers how just being pregnant changed her entire outlook on life – she felt complete. She knew this was what she wanted.

From the day I found out I was pregnant I would put my feet on the floor in the morning when I got out of bed and I would experience this overwhelming feeling of happiness and joy. It wasn't until I experienced a healthy pregnancy that I realised I had been unhappy – it was as if this dark cloud lifted.

Deborah says she had the 'best pregnancy' and that she was the 'happiest, healthiest, most radiant pregnant woman'. She lost the weight she had gained when she was having fertility treatment and she felt healthy enough to work until a few weeks before the date that Will was due. Considering how long she had waited for Will, Deborah wanted to take the right steps to ensure a safe birth. She asked her specialist about having an elective Caesarean. Her specialist favoured her having a natural birth and that is what she had. She finished work on a Friday, her waters broke on a Sunday and Will was born on the Monday – almost three weeks before his due date.

Because it had been such an emotional ride just getting to this point, I was expecting both Phill and I to be quite emotional at the birth. But we were just happy for him to be born. It was quite surreal. I remember looking at Will and thinking, 'You don't know how long I've been waiting for you to arrive.'

During her pregnancy Deborah wrote a journal about her everyday experiences. Her opening paragraph read:

To our unborn child, one day you will know how much trouble your dad and I went through to be parents and have you in our

*life. I love you already and will do so every day for the rest of
my life. All my love, your mother.*

She also collected special treasures for her baby. If she was
at the beach and found an unusual or beautiful shell, she
would bring it home for her unborn son. It was as if she was
willing him into being. Now that he is a toddler, Deborah
still writes letters to Will in which she tells him how she feels
about him, what he is up to in life and how she feels about
being a mother. She says being a mother 'is the ultimate'.
I ask her if it was worth having IVF, but I already know the
answer – absolutely.

> *When you have an overwhelming desire to have a child nothing
> ever takes that feeling away. I think that if you want a child
> and are unfortunate not to be a parent – and there are many
> women who don't conceive using IVF – then that feeling doesn't
> go away if you are 45, 55 or 65. If it is something that you
> wanted, then for the rest of your life there is a part of you that
> will be completely unfulfilled.*

Just as I am starting to think that Will is the ultimate
miracle in Deborah's life, she surprises me by telling me that
since his birth she has had more fertility treatment. She'd had
three more cycles of IVF, none of which were successful. When
I spoke to her in December 2003 she was prepared to make one
last roll of the dice. She had two embryos which she was going
to have implanted in early 2004, after she and Phill returned
from a business trip to New York. This would be her last
attempt at having another child.

I am ready for closure. I will be disappointed if it doesn't work out, but I am 42 and I have been quite consumed by pregnancy for seven years. It is only now that I can sit back and realise how consumed I have been. I didn't feel it at the time I was going through it. I feel blessed that I have a healthy child, and while both myself and my husband want more children, the time has come to put me first.

Is this then one of the key dilemmas of being an older mother – realising you have to forsake any desire for more children because of the biological clock? Or is it that for a woman in her forties, having two children instead of one would be too much to cope with financially, physically and emotionally? It is a complex issue, but Deborah doesn't think it applies only to older women – it's agonising at any age to realise you can't have any more children. There were cumulative reasons for Deborah's decision that the time had come to stop wanting another child.

Your age is a reality that you can't discard and for me it was a key factor. I know that was the reason I had problems getting pregnant, because of my age. This is not the case for everyone but it was with me.

But I also feel that I am at the best part of my life. A woman in her forties has almost reached where she wants to be in her life both personally and often professionally – she has reached a certain fork in the road and it is now a matter of taking a different path or pursuing the same path.

For me it is now about being able to enjoy each day with Will, because he is such a joy, and continuing to appreciate Phill and our marriage as well as my business because it's also part of who I am.

My life has been consumed with having children and I feel that it is now time to make time for myself, whether to do exercise or other things, apart from family.

Deborah says she has been fortunate to be able to make a happy transition between becoming a new mother and returning to work. Soon after Will was born she returned to work three days a week, hiring a nanny to look after her son. When he was a year old she went back to work four days a week. Deborah says having a nanny has made the work–family juggle so much easier as she knows that when she walks out the door, Will is getting the best of care.

I also feel very blessed that I have my own business. This gives me flexibility in my working hours so that if I want to be at the front row of the kindy concert then I can do that. I chose not to work on his birthday – he didn't know any different, but I did. Being able to do these things, to be with him at special times, has made me happier at work.

Deborah also knows she can't afford to miss out on these times because Will may well be her only child. Add to this the fact that he is even more precious because of what she had to go through to bring him into the world. She says Will is like a treasure to her and Phill, and everyone in their inner circle of family and friends feels the same way. She can't help but describe him as a 'miracle' child.

As a successful career woman who almost lost the gamble on

becoming a mother in her forties, what advice does Deborah have for other women who find themselves facing similar decisions about having a child, particularly those women who may need to seek help by having IVF?

My advice to these women is that if they do need IVF they should absolutely do it – and keep going. I spoke to someone recently who was going to start fertility treatment and I had only three words for her: never give up.

I always believed I would have a child. I also felt that I would do whatever I had to do to have a child.

Now, having had Will, I know that a child unites a family. It gives you a sense of family. Before Will there was Phill and me; we were a couple and we loved each other but we were still individuals. Now that Will is here we are a family.

Postscript: By mid-2004 Deborah had not used her two remaining frozen embryos. She still says she wants to use these embryos to try and have another baby. She has had three failed IVF treatments since Will was born. 'Fingers crossed it may happen in the future,' she says. Deborah is reluctant to say if this will be her final attempt at having a second child. 'I feel you always have to have hope,' she says.

Mary-Rose MacColl

author

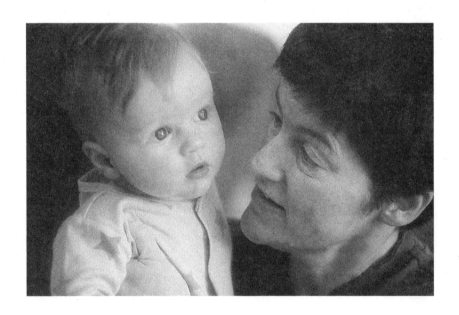

'In my case, being older has made some things easier. I can take a longer view of some things now than I could in my twenties. I'm more realistic about what life has to offer and what I can achieve.'

IT WAS VIRGINIA WOOLF who famously wrote, in her 1928 essay, *A Room of One's Own*, that a woman must have money and a room of her own if she is to write fiction. Perhaps she should have added: 'This is particularly essential for a woman who is also a mother.'

Novelist and mother, Mary-Rose MacColl, 42, has a room of her own, a studio beneath her Brisbane home. Since the birth of her son, Otis, in July 2002, this is where Mary-Rose goes to 'work' three mornings a week, while a babysitter looks after her son.

On weekends, Mary-Rose's husband, David Mayocchi, takes Otis out for a few hours to give Mary-Rose more time to return to her writing life which has seen her produce three novels since 1996. These arrangements are a necessity when there's a toddler in the house. Anyone sitting in on our interview would quickly realise that the utopian vision of a mother working from home, toddler cheerfully playing quietly by her side, has little to do with reality. Otis is 18 months old – an age when children are consumed both by an overwhelming curiosity about the world and the need to have their mother's undivided attention.

An older mother, who after a miscarriage at 40 thought she might not be able to have a child, Mary-Rose has learned to make the best of both worlds. Since giving birth to Otis, she has relaxed her strict approach to writing. She has also found her new life as a mother has overlapped into her fiction in unexpected ways, ensuring a richer creative well for her to draw on.

When Otis was only nine months old and Mary-Rose was being interviewed about her latest novel, *Killing Superman*, she said that 'being a writer requires a simple life; the simpler your life gets the better your writing gets. Otis teaches me a lot about simplicity, just being in the moment and enjoying it.'[1]

Almost ten months later, Mary-Rose still feels that being a writer and an older mother has proved a surprisingly fertile combination.

Having Otis has made me more open to the world. It has also made me less intense about my writing. Next to having a child any experience can seem unimportant. Maybe writing used to give me all my life's meaning and now it doesn't.

Becoming a mother is the most wonderful thing that has ever happened to me. It has changed things completely, and it's not all easy, but the rewards are great.

Having Otis in my life has certainly been better for me, but it's also been better for my writing. Being more relaxed about writing means I feel more free to do what I like. Maybe I'm not so caught up with trying to be the best. I think I can torture my work too much. I don't have the luxury of time to do that now.

Mary-Rose was 41 when she gave birth to Otis. Her husband, David, was 43. They had beeen married for ten years before they became parents. Clearly, having a child has reshaped their lives. No longer just a couple, they've had to forsake the overseas trips and evenings out they had enjoyed over the years for evenings at home looking after Otis.

For Mary-Rose, who has spent much of the past decade focusing on her writing (and having the luxury of time to do so) it must have been a big change to set aside her craft to dedicate herself to motherhood. She is her son's main carer. David works full-time as a manager at a Brisbane educational institution. How, I wondered, did the writer in her cope with this enormous shift in her emotional and creative life, especially when motherhood arrived by the time she had settled into a routine of writing and living?

When I meet her, Mary-Rose appears to have coped very well, perhaps better than she expected, particularly as an older mother whose energies are sapped by age and as a writer with a notorious eye for detail. On a steamy Sunday morning in Brisbane, Mary-Rose tells me that she has just sent her latest manuscript to her agent. The novel, a crime story, about a young girl from a Brisbane political family who becomes involved in armed robbery, was completed after Mary-Rose gave birth to Otis. She already has an idea for another novel, which she hopes to complete this year. In the first year of Otis's life she launched her third novel, *Killing Superman*.

Still, there have been moments over the past eighteen

months which have threatened the fine balance Mary-Rose has created between being a mother and a novelist. She recalls that when she attended the launch of *Killing Superman* in Brisbane, for the first time her mind wasn't on what to wear or what she was going to say in her speech. Instead, baby matters loomed large.

> Killing Superman *was published just before Otis turned one, and I can remember the biggest worry for me at the time was what to do about Otis. The launch was at his sleep time and here I was, with a book coming out, and all I could worry about was how to get Otis to sleep.*

Mary-Rose was in her late twenties when her search for meaning found a focus in writing. The age when some women may start to consider having children, it is also a time when many women have reached a position in their professional life when their hard work is starting to reap rewards. Mary-Rose had established a career in higher education administration when she went back to her childhood love of writing stories. For Mary-Rose, her early to mid-thirties were a time of intense creative development as she started to focus on her writing and had the first of her books published. Children were not yet on the agenda, although the subject did come up with the regularity of a New Year's resolution: 'As David would say, we used to put having children on our list every year. We would say this year we have to decide whether we want to have children.'

However, the years rolled by and the subject of children was gently sidelined by Mary-Rose's growing success as a writer. The daughter of respected Brisbane journalists, Rosemary Lynch and the late Dugald MacColl, Mary-Rose had initially decided she would follow her parents into the newspaper business. She started a cadetship in journalism with Queensland Newspapers in Brisbane, but left to travel. In her early twenties, she worked in a series of jobs, including one in a university as a photocopier operator. She remained in the university sector for the next fifteen years, completing a degree in journalism and eventually working as the executive officer to the Vice-Chancellor at the Queensland University of Technology (QUT).

I had a lot of different jobs in my early twenties. Then I got hooked into corporate life at QUT, working long hours and feeling very much part of the institutional culture. Looking back now, I'm glad I wasn't married and thinking about having children. I don't think I could have been a mother then, not at that age. In my early twenties, I don't think I would have managed. It's such an all-encompassing experience, especially in those early months. I'd have been overwhelmed. And then once my career got going, I'd have been forced to take time out which I wouldn't have wanted to do.

Having children has been a choice for my generation. No one pressured us to have children, and contraception was a fact of life. It was different for my mother's generation. When she had children, she gave up work. Having children was what you did once you got married, and then you left work and cared for the children.

In the early 1990s, while still at QUT, Mary-Rose channelled her creative instincts as a writer into her first book, a crime novel called *No Safe Place*. It was runner-up in the

Australian Vogel Literary Award and published in 1996. Her next book, *Angels in the Architecture*, was published in 1999, followed by *Killing Superman* in July 2003. As well as her writing her novels, Mary-Rose has also taught writing (she holds a Masters degree in creative writing from the University of Queensland) and chaired the 1998 Brisbane Writers Festival.

When she was almost 38, Mary-Rose decided it was time to stop thinking about whether to have children and start trying to conceive. Initially she wasn't concerned about her ability to get pregnant because she says she had not understood the full impact of age on a woman's fertility.

> *I knew fertility rates dropped off with age, but I just thought that meant that some women weren't fertile any more. I didn't know that it affected all women. The first I knew that it might not be a cinch was when I went to my doctor and said, 'David and I want to have a baby.'*
>
> *My doctor said, 'Okay, come back and see me if you are not pregnant within a few months.' I don't think she was trying to panic me, but she was trying to make me aware that there is a problem with women and age and fertility.*
>
> *And I can understand her doing that. Doctors must feel pressured in these situations because if women aren't made aware of the facts, they can't make informed decisions about their lives.*
>
> *I think we gloss over the facts about age and fertility. Maybe in my case I'd been ambivalent about having children so I didn't make a point of finding out the facts.*

Mary-Rose had decided that she did not want to use any kind of fertility treatment if she failed to fall pregnant naturally.

She says she did not want to use Clomid, a drug that encourages ovulation, which can be prescribed by a GP and is also used by fertility clinics before a woman has more advanced treatment such as IVF.

> *I wanted to be open to having a baby, but I didn't want to interfere with the process. It had taken me a long time to decide I wanted to have a child. Having decided, I wanted to let nature take its course.*
>
> *At the time, of course, I had no idea that getting pregnant might be difficult. At the start, I thought we'd get pregnant in the first month. When that didn't happen, I was surprised. It ended up taking over a year, and by then I really wanted a baby . . . You know how if you want something and you don't get it then you want it even more.*
>
> *Then I had a miscarriage which was very difficult to cope with. It was very early in the pregnancy – about seven to eight weeks. I don't know how women cope with later miscarriages. Your body and mind are all geared towards this baby you've conceived, and then it's gone. I was terribly upset.*
>
> *By then I'd done some reading about age and fertility and I realised I might never have a child. I still didn't want to use any drugs or pursue IVF. I decided to get on with life on the basis that I wouldn't have a child. If a child came along, okay, and if not, that would be okay too.*
>
> *What really helped me then was getting used to the idea that I could still have a life without kids. I had to stop worrying about what the future would bring and start living in the moment. I do yoga and swim which are good for getting me back into the present.*

Any time I wondered about whether I might be pregnant or not, I used to visualise a baby floating out to sea in a basket and wave it off.

We got on with life, bought a new car, a little Holden that's hopeless for a family, and a two-level townhouse with a million safety hazards and no yard.

About six months after her miscarriage, Mary-Rose fell pregnant with Otis.

One of four children, Mary-Rose had many friends who'd had children. So she'd had quite a bit to do with other people's children – but not a lot to do with babies. As a result, having an infant in the house was a shock. Besides, she notes, 'having your own child is completely different' to being with other people's children. Being an older mother, she says, has a downside in that she doesn't have as much energy as she would if she was younger. This made it hard, she says, dealing with the sleepless nights that can be a new parent's lot well into the first two years of a child's life.

I'm also a complete control freak, which probably gets worse with age. I can remember bursting into tears when Otis was a baby simply because he didn't go to sleep when I thought he would. I've had to learn to be more flexible. Otis is an excellent teacher.

For Mary-Rose, the upside of being an older mother has been a patience that comes with maturity, as well as a sense of perspective.

In my case, being older has made some things easier. I can take a longer view of some things now than I could in my twenties. I'm more realistic about what life has to offer and what I can achieve.

I also have a longer view of what a career offers. In my twenties, I worked really hard at QUT as a corporate writer and then changed careers and became a full-time fiction writer. I loved doing both things and would not have given them up easily.

If I'd had Otis back then, I would have had to miss a lot of his young life or miss my work. I wasn't ready to make that kind of choice.

I loved my work at QUT and I love writing. Because I changed career, my early thirties were a crucial time in establishing myself as a writer. If I hadn't been able to do that, I'm not sure I'd feel as happy as I do now.

At the same time, I know that a career isn't everything. It doesn't give my life all its meaning.

Even so, Mary-Rose needed to find a way to continue with her writing once Otis was born. But how to cope with writing when you have a baby in the house?

When he was really little, I'd sit with him in a sling while I typed onto the laptop. Then when he got a bit bigger, he'd sleep on the floor of the lounge while I worked. I can remember dragging him around the room to get him out of a patch of sun which moved across the floor during the day. I'd also write early in the morning after his first feed, and then sleep later in the day when he slept.

Mary-Rose drew on the advice of friends and colleagues, many of whom had children. A newspaper reporter asked her about the juggle between work and writing when Otis was just over a year old and Mary-Rose recalled some advice a colleague had given her. The advice was 'to take a year off when you have Otis. If you don't feel like doing any writing and you are really enjoying time with Otis, just enjoy it and do that. Don't let anyone make you feel that you're not a proper person because you are not doing anything but looking after Otis. If, on the other hand, you are feeling "antsy" arrange to have enough care for him that you can write.'

> *It was good advice. I've kept swimming and writing ever since Otis was born. I can see how easy it would be to give yourself up completely with the neediness of a child.*

Mary-Rose has recently hired a babysitter to come into her home to look after Otis. She also took the Virginia Woolf option and set up a room of her own so that she had a proper workplace to go to when she wanted to write. She had to temper a fastidious streak which often emerges in her writing in the form of meticulous research and attention to detail.

> *With Otis, I am a lot more focused where writing is concerned. I used to worry too much about writing. I'd spend hours and hours sitting at the computer forcing myself to write or taking my psychological pulse and wondering, 'Do I have anything meaningful to say today?'*
>
> *Now I have less time to write. As soon as the babysitter arrives or Otis is asleep, it is a case of get to the computer and get some writing done before he wakes up! It's a nice change to the pace of my days.*

Becoming a mother has made Mary-Rose consider what life was like for her own mother, who was in her mid-twenties when she had the first of her four children. Like many women of Rosemary Lynch's generation, the beginning of her life as a mother was also the end of her life as a working woman. Age had nothing to do with it – this was just the way of the world in the 1950s and 1960s. Child care was not an option and her husband was working full-time.

Having Otis and seeing the impact he has had on my life has helped me start to understand what it must have been like for my mother. She was a journalist, and a really good journalist, and she had to quit her career to have her kids. She stayed home with them. As I was getting older I was already starting to think about what it was like for her to do that, but having Otis has made me feel an incredible kind of empathy.

She was in her mid-twenties when she had her first child. There were four of us, and she was mostly alone. Dad would go to work at 4pm every day and come home at 1am and then sleep in until after we went to school. I don't know how she didn't go insane. Most days I can't wait for David to get home.

I think I am lucky to have been born when I was, and to have been able to have a career and a child and have some sort of life of my own. I am very lucky also because David is such a devoted father, and it is not just something that he feels he should do. He can't wait to come home and see Otis. And Otis adores him.

At 44, David is an older father and a very happy one. He loves his son. However, it was interesting to hear Mary-Rose's

account of how she and David had often talked around the issue
of parenthood.

> *David always said he'd go along with what I wanted, but if
> I hadn't wanted a child he'd have been happy not to have one,
> he said. People would say to me that David would just love
> being a father. They were right. What surprised me was how
> much he loves Otis and how much he loves being a father.*

Before Otis was born David didn't feel the need to be a
father. I wondered if Mary-Rose was worried about this, particularly since her own father had worked long hours and hadn't
been very involved in his children's young lives. Also, *Killing
Superman* was about a troubled relationship between a son and
his father. Was she worried about David's ability to be a father?

> *Actually, I think he was more worried than I was. He was
> worried that he wouldn't enjoy it. If I was surprised it was only
> at how quickly David came on board, within a few days of Otis
> being born.*
>
> *David was worried about being a father but I don't think he
> is now. I think he'd happily stay home with Otis if my writing
> made enough money for us to survive that way.*
>
> *Otis thinks David is the ant's pants at the moment. They
> have a great time together. It's been good for me and has freed me
> up to do things for myself.*

I ask Mary-Rose if she has thought of having more children.
Of course, she says, but to tell the truth, she is not yet sure if
she will or she won't.

I really don't know. If I was ten years younger, I'd probably try to have more children, but if we are going to have another baby then you have some big issues to think about, including those ever-declining fertility rates and increased risk of Down syndrome.

Also, there is the danger of not enjoying what you already have. Her personal life is richer with Otis and she has another book to write. 'I'm happy with my life right now,' Mary-Rose says. 'It just keeps getting better.'

Sandra McLean

journalist and author

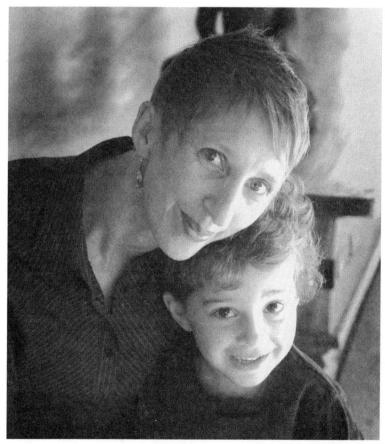

JUSTINE WALPOLE

'People say that children change your life —
they lie. Children take over your life, turn it
upside down and leave you to sort out what
matters.'

UNTIL MY SON Hamish was born I never really questioned the way I had lived my life. But it was only a few nights after his birth, when I was still in hospital and experiencing one of those surreal pre-dawn breastfeeds, that I realised how odd life can be. I mean, isn't it crazy that, at 17, I thought I knew enough about the world to leave home and move to a new city — and yet, here I was at 38 and pretty much clueless about one of life's most basic tasks, looking after a baby. Just as unsettling was the new way in which I looked at my mother. She came to the rescue in those first blurry days when we brought Hamish home from hospital. During this time it dawned on me what a challenge her own life as a new mum must have been — and how different an experience it had been to my own.

My mum was 20 when she gave birth to my sister, the first of her three children. It was 1957 and she had been teaching for two years after a year of study at teachers college in Brisbane. It was a short course because the post-war baby boom meant that there was a shortage of teachers. Even so, my mother could not claim her own superannuation and when she left her job to have my sister she was forced to quit. She told me that, in the late 1950s and early 1960s, female teachers were put off at the end of each year as they were considered temporary employees, expected to leave the profession eventually to start families.

When I was 20, I was working as a cadet journalist for a metropolitan newspaper in Brisbane, living in a share house and attempting to finish a Bachelor of Arts degree at the University of Queensland. The very thought of having a child at that age now makes me feel a little queasy. I was young, irresponsible and completely ignorant of anything to do with children. I marvel now at my mother who, by the age of 25, had three children under five. Yet hers is not an unusual story for the times. Back then I would have been the unusual one. Quentin Bryce, the governor of Queensland, once told me in an interview that she had been unique in her neighbourhood in Brisbane in the 1960s because she was a working mum. She wasn't ostracised – quite the opposite, with offers of support flowing from friendly neighbours who must have marvelled at this woman who was studying law (she became the first woman in Queensland called to the bar) and raising children. By the time she turned 30, Bryce had five children under seven.

Interestingly, a few years before my interview with her, Bryce had remarked to a journalist writing a story on only children, that the pupils at Women's College at the University of Sydney, where she was then principal, never talked about children or becoming mothers. 'Speaking to young women here, you simply never run into any who are very pro-children,' she told the journalist.

No surprise to me. As a young woman, I – like my friends – was petrified of getting pregnant. We all tried our darndest to avoid it. The abortion debate was running hot, particularly in Queensland where it had the power to divide communities and push governments into political oblivion. We were all far more aware of the downside of having children than any upside. I can't recall anyone telling me how wonderful it was to have children. I can't even recall anyone talking about children and I doubt this has changed much among the 20 year olds of today who want and need to experience independence.

We were the new generation of feminists – sisters doing it for themselves, as Eurythmics singer Annie Lennox told us. We were focused on things such as work and travel, which seemed far more important than family. We knew more about those things. We didn't know about motherhood nor were we encouraged to find out. Not that it was always that way – I can remember doing Mothercare lessons at high school in Townsville, where we were taught about the different stages of pregnancy, how to put on a nappy and the best way to nurse a baby. I also remember that these classes were aimed at preparing us just in case the unspeakable happened and we became – horror of horrors – teenage mothers.

Through my twenties and into my thirties I didn't think much about being a mother. It was a concept as unfamiliar to me as life on Mars. My female friends didn't talk about it either. We were hardly sitting around yearning to breastfeed or play catch in the park with our beloved offspring.

However, in the mid-1990s things started to change. Suddenly one friend fell pregnant, then another. Another friend had twins. An old friend who was living in the UK had a boy. These women were about my age, in their mid- to late-thirties.

I can't say how it happened – call it osmosis – but my husband Phil and I decided that, er, maybe we should, um, think about, gee, having a child. We had bought a house and we'd traversed the globe several times in the eight years we'd been together. My job had given me many years of satisfaction, working in Brisbane, Sydney and London. At the time I was the arts editor of the *Courier-Mail* in Brisbane. Looking back it was an exceedingly casual decision. I went off the contraceptive pill and we hit the sheets.

Great idea, but nothing happened. For six months we tried, but I did not conceive. Was there a problem? Off we went to my doctor, who suggested we kept trying for a few more months. I was about to celebrate my thirty-seventh birthday. If I knew then what I do now about the way fertility plummets as you progress through your thirties I would not have been so relaxed.

Even at 37 I was playing with pretty tight odds and was facing an uphill battle to conceive. Anxious to make conception easier, I read books about body temperature and cervical mucus acting as fertility barometers. I was given a lipstick-like contraption that was supposed to help me identify when I was ovulating. It involved putting saliva on the top of the lipstick and hitting a button that shone a light on the saliva. If a fern-like pattern materialised, then I was ovulating or about to ovulate and it was time to have sex. For weeks I saw nothing but a sludge of saliva.

So off we went, back to my GP, who advised me to take a low dose of Clomid, a drug which encourages ovulation. She also suggested my husband have a sperm test so we could identify the problematic party. I never thought Phil would agree to this, but bless him, he did, travelling across Brisbane, sperm in jar, with as much dignity as the situation would allow. It turned out that his sperm were fine, so the problem lay with me.

I took Clomid and for a few months nothing happened. We decided to live our lives normally and not get too worried about the fact we were having trouble conceiving. I had made up my mind that I was not going to have IVF because I wasn't prepared to undergo any invasive treatment. Also, I had a fatalistic attitude to getting pregnant – if it didn't happen then it wasn't meant to be. I hoped I would be able to build a philosophical structure to help me cope with not being a mother. Fortunately, Phil felt the same way. In hindsight, knowing how much joy and wonder Hamish has brought into my life, I wonder how we would have lived with such an outcome – and if we would have changed our minds about IVF.

In September 1999, we went to Canberra to visit my sister. I had been tempted to toss away my lipstick ovulation marker but decided to give it one last go in Canberra. It was springtime, heck you never know. I woke up on the Sunday morning of our visit, a little bleary-eyed from the night before, and looked, for the umpteenth time, at my saliva. I saw fern patterns.

A few weeks later I missed my period. I went to the doctor. Yes, I was five weeks pregnant. My immediate reaction was panic. We were going to Bali for a holiday in the following fortnight. I can remember walking up the road back to work telling Phil on my mobile phone I was pregnant and then calling my parents and telling them the news as well.

It was a truly surreal moment. A train rumbled past me as I stood at the level crossing. The world appeared the same but I knew it had changed irrevocably for me at that moment.

Of course I didn't consider myself an older mother and my doctor encouraged me to keep working, exercising and doing the things I enjoyed. This included travelling and we ended up going to Bali and also to Hong Kong five months later. By the time he was born Hamish was a very well-travelled young man.

At the time of writing he is three and a half years old. People say that children change your life – they lie. Children take over your life, turn it upside down and leave you to sort out what matters.

When I fell pregnant I agreed to take six months maternity leave. I received six weeks paid leave under the Media Entertainment Arts Alliance Award. We had saved enough money to keep us going for a few more months without my wage. But when the six months was up I knew I could not go back to work. How could I leave a six-month-old baby in day care? So I applied for another six months unpaid leave.

During that year away from work with Hamish my world shrank in some ways and expanded in others. Being a stay-at-home mum opened my eyes to another world that existed parallel to my former life as a swinging career gal. I went to shopping malls and marvelled at the crowds of people, mainly mums and their children. I spent rewarding time with my mother and mother-in-law, all of us brought closer through the new baby in our lives. Work floated off into another world but, while it became a blur, I felt it still had a role in my life. I also felt that since I had successfully given birth and managed to keep my child alive and healthy to the age of one, returning to work would be a breeze.

After all, I had survived sleepless nights, mastered breast-feeding, worked out how to put the pram up and down – and Phil and I were still married. Workplace politics would be a cinch. Of course, I was wrong. The guts and glory of mother-hood meant little to the people who had been encased in the working world while I had been away for a year.

When the year was up I returned to work four days a week. Only a few weeks later I was removed from my position as arts editor and put into the writing pool. I felt it was a demotion, though it was not described as that, of course. However, everyone in newspapers knows that being a writer is less influ-ential than being an editor. I didn't lose any pay, but it hurt professionally and personally. I felt betrayed. Looking back, I should have been angrier and more outspoken about how I felt about the 'restructure'.

At the time, I just couldn't face any more drama. Our lives were precarious enough – Hamish had started going to day care, he had been ill with ear infections, a full night's sleep was still a rarity. We didn't need more stress in our lives.

At that point, I wondered if being an older mother was really much of an advantage in the workplace. After all, my experi-ence and savvy had not saved me from losing the job I believed was rightfully mine. Being older, however, did eventually give me the emotional strength to counter this disappointment with a realisation that there is more to life than work, that I was working in a position with less stress and could enjoy more time with Hamish. Even so, the experience made me angry and I felt that the change had happened for the wrong reasons. Also, I believed it had not been handled at all well by my employers.

These days I am more relaxed about work and more confident about my abilities. It's probably no accident that this newfound calm is paralleled by a more serene environment at home now that I have learned a lot more about how to cope with the challenges of having a child.

I still feel strongly that more should be done by employers to cater for new working mothers. For all the talk by governments desperate to reverse Australia's declining fertility rate and encourage women to have children and stay at home to look after them, there is little pressure put on big business to help out in the simplest of ways, such as encouraging new mothers to work from home, having a better attitude to flexible working hours or building childcare facilities within the place of work. At the time of writing, there was no universal paid maternity leave in Australia; indeed John Howard's federal government is actively opposed to such a scheme, even though federal public servants in Australia are entitled to paid maternity leave.

Parenthood raises many questions – and I'm not just talking about how on earth a toddler seems to innately know what a vegetable looks like. For older mothers there is one pressing question that is most difficult to answer: when, indeed if, to have another child? Just hours after I had given birth to Hamish my obstetrician remarked, jokingly (I think), how it would be lovely to see me back in the hospital for baby number two. Having just had an episiotomy, I wondered if this amazing woman who had calmly helped deliver my baby was some kind of sadist. Certainly her timing could have been better!

I had just come out of a seventeen-hour labour and had been handed some rather large, boat-like pads to stem post-labour bleeding. Nobody had told me about this part of childbirth but I realised then that from then on I would have to deal with whatever came my way. After childbirth my feelings were intense. I wanted to freeze this moment in my life so I wrote down what had happened the night before; how the labour pains had started at about 7.30pm over a bowl of pumpkin and coriander soup; how, as the pain intensified, the midwife had suggested I have a hot shower and Phil had yelled at her that it was bloody obvious something a little stronger was needed. Finally, around 5am the anaesthetist arrived to give me an epidural, chatting about where he could get the best bread at this time of day. After the epidural it was strangely pleasant as we chatted inanely with the midwife, who I realised I knew from a local dance class. Finally at midday my obstetrician, Fiona, arrived and with the statement, 'Let's get this baby born', everyone got down to business.

After a lot of pushing, and not much to show for it, Fiona decided on a vacuum extraction. Two more contractions and more desperate pushing (I was starting to get worried at this point) and Hamish was born at 1.43pm on 21 July 2000, weighing 3.2 kilos. Phil, who is squeamish at the sight of a needle, was there for the entire labour, although he admits he watched a game of tennis out the window when the going got tough. I can't remember labour being traumatic or terribly painful – perhaps it was and I have simply blotted it out. I do recall, though, from the moment I got to the hospital, a sense of inevitability, that there was no other way to do this but one step at a time. When Hamish was put to my breast minutes after he was born, it was both strange and familiar. I said, 'How bizarre', and Fiona told Phil to kiss me – and he did.

I am frequently asked by people when I will have another child. They don't mean to pry – it is the obvious question. I silently wonder every time: 'Don't they know I'm over 40?'. Having waited until I was 38 to have Hamish, I've made it tougher to have a second child. The biological clock is ticking loudly now that I am into my fifth decade.

At the moment, however, both Phil and I are happy to say: once is enough. We have a wonderful child in Hamish, so why push our luck?

When I was trying to get pregnant in my late thirties I was blithely ignorant of the risks involved in having a baby later in life: the higher chance of miscarriage, of having a baby with Down syndrome. I didn't know that my fertility was plummeting, which was a good thing as I didn't panic when I failed to fall pregnant immediately. Now that I know all this I am much more thoughtful about having another baby. I am not sure if I want to put myself in a position where I end up wanting something that I might not be able to have.

Also, if we had another child we would have to move house and in this day and age, with hefty mortgages and rising interest rates (not to mention changing suburbs and maybe not being able to find a day care place for Hamish), this is not something to be taken lightly!

Sadly, though, single children are still considered somehow unfortunate, even in the twenty-first century. This is a shame. Perhaps we need to rethink our attitude toward this. Having one baby has brought me more joy than I had ever anticipated.

In writing this book I have learned that there is no one way to approach the issue of late babies. Every woman has done it her own way. For some, the fact they were older and more advanced in their careers gave them a valuable flexibility so they could work around their children's lives. For others, age provided them with the wisdom to know what was best for themselves, their child and their relationships. There are no rules when it comes to being a mother and making your life work around this amazing experience, just as there is no right time in a woman's life to have her first child. I find it uplifting that in this often over-managed world, where it's easy to feel like part of a production line, there is a whole lot of room for individuals to work out a way of life that suits them. For me, the door to this room was the one with the baby picture on it. It may have taken me a while to find it, but better late than never, I say.

The trend to older motherhood

The biological clock is ticking, but are women listening? It is a fact of Australian life that first-time mums are getting older. According to the Australian Bureau of Statistics (ABS), the median age of mothers in 2002 was 30.2 – the highest on record. Twenty-five years ago the median age of first-time mothers was 24.[1]

The corollary of this trend to delaying childbirth is the accelerating decrease in the number of births to women aged in their twenties. According to the ABS, in 2002 women aged 30–34 had the highest birth rate with 111 births per 1000 women. This compared to a dramatic slump in births among women under 29. Over the past twenty years, the birth rate among this age group has almost halved from 104 babies per 1000 women in 1982 to 56 babies in 2002.[2]

The dramatic drop in the number of women giving birth in

their twenties is a key factor in Australia's falling fertility rate. Clearly, the gains being made by older women can't keep up with the drop in the birth rate among younger women, even though women aged 35–39 have increased their rate of giving birth since 1982, from 25.6 births per 1000 to 42.2 per 1000 in 2002.

The great fertility droop

So statistics tell us that women are delaying childbirth until later in life. They also tell us that women are having fewer children. In 2002 the fertility rate (the number of children a woman would bear over her lifetime) was 1.75 babies per woman. This is half what it was at the peak of the so-called 'baby boom' in 1961 when it reached 3.5 babies per woman. The rate started to droop after the boom and by 1976 it had fallen to 2.1.[3]

Our baby-making rate has not only stalled but is showing worrying signs of declining further as more Australian women and their partners decide not to have children.

According to ABS 2002 estimates, about 25 per cent of women currently in their reproductive years are likely to remain childless.[4]

This decline in fertility hasn't come as a surprise to demographers. In general, the trend was started in the 1960s and 1970s by the availability of the contraceptive pill and the advent of feminism, and was then fuelled by changing social conditions such as late marriages, higher education levels and the desire for more choice in life. Economic recession also played a part. These influences have been evident for almost twenty years. But, if we consider this trend from a historical perspective, we can see this is not the first time Australia has experienced a decline in fertility rates.

War and poverty can wreak havoc on a woman's desire to procreate, as well as her ability to find a suitable partner. In the first four decades of the twentieth century Australian women had to endure both. First there was World War I which took thousands of virile young men out of the breeding equation. Then there was the Great Depression when unemployment, lack of money and not much hope forced the idea of family well onto the back burner. In 1934, at the height of the Great Depression, fertility levels fell to 2.1 babies per woman.[5]

Women who had deferred childbearing during those tough Depression years began to have children again in the late 1930s. This pattern repeated itself after World War II and fertility increased through the 1950s, peaking in 1961, when the fertility rate reached an impressive 3.5 babies per woman. But these fertile times were not to last and the decline was swift. By 1966, only five years after the peak, the fertility rate had fallen to 2.9. Demographers tend to put the blame for this emphatic dip in fertility levels on the introduction of oral contraception to Australia in 1961 which enabled women to more easily and effectively control their reproductive future.

Once the trend started, it didn't stop. By 1976 fertility rates had fallen to below the official replacement level of 2.1. By the start of the twenty-first century, Australia's fertility rate had halved from 3.5 to 1.75 in a period of just forty years.

Fertility and survival

So what if our fertility levels are falling? Why the worried looks from policymakers and politicians? Surely, fewer people means less pressure on precious resources and the environment? Well, yes . . . and no. The problem is that a declining birth rate is a major factor contributing to population ageing. This has important social and financial implications for the way families function and for society generally. If the workforce shrinks, then health-care and income support costs increase.[6]

As a result, more pressure is put on the government to provide for the elderly. But an ageing population means there are too few new taxpayers to prop up pensions, health-care and economic growth. Hence the concern among political parties over this country's falling fertility levels. More demand on government coffers means more taxes and that is not a vote-winning strategy for any party. Also, without steady population growth, economic growth can stall. And there are major implications for age-based social institutions such as schools and, in particular, universities, which could experience reduced demand for places.

However, declining fertility levels can reflect positive changes. These include better education and a wider range of choices for women. As noted by David De Vaus, a senior research adviser at the Australian Institute of Family Studies, it would be wrong and unacceptable to reduce opportunities for women with a view to increasing fertility. The role of policy, he says, should be to enable couples to have the number of children they choose.[7]

What is a late baby anyway?

Clinically, late babies are defined as those born to women over 35 years of age. When I was pregnant, at 38, my obstetrician joked that medically, I would be called an 'elderly primi-gravida', an older woman who is pregnant for the first time. The other term that is often used is 'elderly primiparae', which refers to an older woman giving birth for the first time. Doctors can take their pick, but these terms sound more like a reference to a stick insect than a pregnant woman. The word 'elderly' sounds ungainly and insulting to today's older mother who considers herself youthful in mind, body and spirit.

However, these terms are more than just labels. They are used by medical staff to designate the special status of older women; because having children after the age of 35 is commonly believed to be a risk to the health of the mother and the baby.[8]

It is from this age that some women may find it hard to get pregnant, and the risks of both miscarriage and genetic abnormalities increases. Mind you, the age at which a woman is termed 'elderly' by health professionals has changed: almost fifteen years ago a woman having a child in her early thirties would have been described as elderly. However, socially speaking, 35 has become the new 30. And there is a distinct possibility this will change again in the not too distant future, according to Queensland University of Technology Associate Professor Karen Thorpe, a psychologist who is also a co-author of *Older Mothers: Conception, Pregnancy and Birth After 35*.

She says that 40 may soon be the age when pregnant women will fall into the 'elderly' category. This is due to a combination of factors. More efficient diagnostic tests, such as chorionic villus sampling and amniocentesis can reduce the risk of an older mother giving birth to a child with a genetic abnormality. Also, an increased level of fitness among women today may reduce the incidence of health risks that can reduce fertility.

These include smoking and being overweight or underweight. Also, it is becoming more of a social norm to be an older mother. Society is more willing to accept that women are having babies later in life. This will lead, Thorpe believes, to an adjustment in society's attitude to what constitutes a 'late' baby.

Does age really matter?

Unfortunately, yes. The statistics may vary by a few percentage points, but talk to any fertility expert, gynaecologist or obstetrician and they will tell you that older women will find it harder to get pregnant and their pregnancies will be riskier. Manager Marian Hudson found out the hard way that age does matter when it comes to making babies – she was told that her inability to fall pregnant after IVF was because of age-related infertility.

Dr Wendy Cox, a leading Sydney obstetrician whose practice deals increasingly with women over 35, says that she sees many women who have managed to beat the sobering statistics on age-related infertility. Still, she has this to say about having babies and getting older: 'If it is really important for you to have children then do it before you are 35. Why? Because of the way a woman's fertility falls.'

According to Professor Michael Chapman, medical director of IVF Australia and a professor of obstetrics at the University of NSW, women are most fertile from the age of 18 through to their mid-twenties. From their mid-twenties, their fertility begins a gradual decline, which gathers speed in their early thirties, accelerates into their late thirties and, by their mid-forties, has virtually disappeared across the horizon. As he puts it: 'The slippery slope, when it comes to fertility, begins after 35.'

Hence what is commonly referred to as the biological clock or body clock – which starts to sound like Big Ben by the time women are in their late thirties and early forties.

According to the US Centers for Disease Control, once a woman celebrates her forty-second birthday, the chances of her having a baby using her own eggs, even with advanced medical help, are less than 10 per cent.[9] Without medical help you can halve that percentage. Similarly, in her book, *Baby Hunger: The New Battle for Motherhood*, economist Sylvia Ann Hewlett, paints a bleak picture for women over 35 hoping to get pregnant. She quotes figures from the Mayo Clinic, a leading research and treatment facility in the United States, indicating that fertility drops 20 per cent after the age of 30, 50 per cent after the age of 35 and 95 per cent after the age of 40. Also, while 72 per cent of 28-year-old women get pregnant after trying for a year, only 24 per cent of 38-year-olds do.[10]

Are these figures applicable in Australia? Professor Chapman says, in general, yes they are. His research and his clinical experience indicate that age-related infertility is particularly problematic for women in their very early forties whom he says have a 5 per cent chance of falling pregnant each time they ovulate. This falls to about 1 per cent for a woman who is over 45. For women aged between 35 and 40, the chance of falling pregnant is estimated at about 10 to 15 per cent each cycle.

Other factors affecting fertility

Getting pregnant at any time in life is like the roll of a dice. Chance and circumstance are major players, even for a 20-year-old woman. According to IVF Australia's Professor Chapman, a healthy young woman aged in her early twenties still only has a 25 per cent chance of getting pregnant each cycle.

As well as age-related infertility, there are other factors which can make it hard for a woman to fall pregnant. These include body weight – being too fat or too thin can affect a woman's chances of pregnancy; smoking; and individual health issues such as instances of sexually transmitted diseases like chlamydia, or the presence of fibroids, pelvic infections or endometriosis.

Risks of older motherhood

Older women find it harder to get pregnant: they also face increased risk of miscarriage as well as higher chances of their child having a genetic abnormality.

In 2002, *Time* magazine published an article which quoted sobering figures from the US Centers for Disease Control regarding miscarriage rates among older women. According to these figures, at 20 the risk of miscarriage is about 9 per cent; it doubles to 18 per cent by 35, then doubles again by the time a woman reaches her early forties. By the time a woman reaches her mid-forties, she has a 53 per cent chance of miscarrying.[11]

Professor Chapman explains that the risk of miscarriage is especially high in women over 40 as up to half their eggs can be chromosomally abnormal, causing the foetus to abort.

But if the mother carries the child to term, the baby may be born with a chromosomal disorder such as Down syndrome or two other conditions, Patau's syndrome and Edward's syndrome, which are much more severe and generally result in death during infancy. According to the National Association for

Down Syndrome in the United Kingdom, a 20-year-old woman has a 1 in 1340 chance of having a baby born with Down syndrome; this figure climbs to 1 in 400 for a 35-year-old woman; 1 in 180 for a 38-year-old woman; 1 in 60 for a 42-year-old woman and 1 in 20 for a 46-year-old.

As well as the chance of a chromosomal disorder, an increased risk of foetal death and increased stillbirth rates have also been reported in women over 35.

The precise reason for the increase in chromosomal abnormalities with the age of the mother is not known. There has been a suggestion that women's eggs are not all perfect and those that are defective are ovulated later in a woman's life. Also, the eggs of an older woman have experienced a longer period of potentially adverse environmental exposures, which may damage a once-perfect egg.[12]

Research has also suggested that hormonal changes which occur later in a woman's reproductive life may influence the process of ovulation causing an 'over-ripening' of the eggs.

Why age matters

It's all about eggs. Prevailing scientific thought states that when a woman is born she comes into the world with all her eggs – several hundred thousand – stored in her ovaries. Each month, after puberty, the ovaries release eggs and the supply is gradually depleted until it ends with menopause, which generally occurs between 45 and 55.

There are no second orders. When the eggs run out – tough. If they are not up to scratch – ditto.

Herein lies the danger in considering fertility treatment the answer to all the pregnancy woes of older women. True, reproductive medicine has made great leaps since the world's first test-tube baby, Louise Brown, was born using in-vitro fertilisation in 1978. It can work wonders for a woman in her late twenties whose fallopian tubes are blocked or for a woman in her early thirties whose husband has a low sperm count. However, it continues to grapple with the enigma that is the egg and its role in infertility in older women.

And the egg could be more of an enigma than previously thought following the intriguing discoveries this year of researchers in the United States. Their research in to how eggs are created could turn on its head the century-old doctrine that females are born with a fixed supply of eggs. The researchers at the Harvard Medical School found that the problem with age-related infertility in women might lie in the stem cells that make new eggs. They found that female mice produced new eggs well into adulthood and the researchers also isolated stems cells which they believe develop into new eggs. If women can make new eggs, the researchers argued, then it also means a way could be found to stimulate this production until late in life. 'If these findings hold up in humans, all theories about the aging of the female reproductive system will have to be revisited,' said Jonathan Tilly, who led the research team at Harvard. Australian doctors described the discovery as 'provocative' and admitted it would 'affect the way we think about female fertility fairly profoundly'.[13]

The research results at Harvard Medical School are remarkable, however, the scientists do not yet know if they apply to humans. Women in the twenty-first century still have to live with the current scientific dogma that says even if 40 might be the new 30; age is still defenceless against Mother Nature. No matter how fit and fabulous a woman may look even at 45, her eggs, biologically speaking, are old.

This is why sheer willpower and diet will never get older women over the line in the fertility race. Yet many of them persist in believing they can cheat the clock. According to a fertility awareness survey carried out by the American Infertility Association in 2001, 39 per cent of respondents thought fertility began to drop at 40 – the correct answer was 27.[14]

A similar survey was undertaken in New South Wales in 2003 by the Family Planning Association Health. It surveyed women aged from 35 to 55 and showed they believed that women had a 62 per cent chance of pregnancy each year in their early 40s (the reality is more like 5 to 10 per cent) and a 48 per cent chance in their late 40s (it is more like 1 per cent). Many had no idea that women aged 40 are, on average, only half as fertile as those aged 25. 'There seems to be a misconception around conception, which makes women think the risk of getting pregnant is very high,' Dr Christine Read, coordinator of medical services at Family Planning Association Health, told the media at the time. 'There is also social pressure, particularly in metropolitan areas, for women to be achievers before they start to think about having a family.'[15]

Older but not wiser to fertility treatment

Since the first IVF baby was born in 1978, assisted reproductive technology (ART) has helped thousands of parents worldwide have children. But these successes must be balanced against ART's many failures, often because of age-related infertility.

According to IVF Australia, the success rate, called the 'take-home baby' rate, will vary between 5 and 50 per cent per attempt or cycle. The figure depends on the woman's age, the number of eggs retrieved, the number that are fertilised (dependent also upon the sperm), the number of embryos transferred and the state of the uterus.

In fact, age is particularly crucial when considering success rates with ART. A chart posted by IVF Australia on its website shows that for women aged between 22 and 34 there is a 50.4 per cent success rate in falling pregnant and delivering a healthy child using IVF. For women aged between 34 and 39, there is a 38.2 per cent success rate. This rate drops dramatically to 15 per cent for women aged between 39 and 44 years.[16]

The graph also reveals the increasing risk of miscarriage with age. About 10 per cent of women in the youngest age group, who fell pregnant, miscarried. But by the time a woman hits 40, the miscarriage rate rises to almost 50 per cent.

And age has a number of other effects on the success of IVF treatment. The number of eggs collected is lower in older women and the quality of the embryos (fertilised eggs) also decreases. As a result, higher doses of hormones are required for older women and there is also a higher risk of not proceeding to egg collection due to poor response to these drugs.

Professor Robert Jansen, medical director of Sydney IVF, looked at the relationship between a woman's age and her hopes of success using IVF in a paper published in the *Medical Journal of Australia* in 2003. Aware of the increasing pressure on IVF to give older women successful pregnancies, Dr Jansen wanted to find out more about the effect of age on the likelihood of a live birth from IVF.

He based his research on all IVF patients (median age 36) who attended a private IVF clinic in Sydney between 1 January 1998, and 31 December, 1998, and had embryo placements performed up to 30 June, 2001.

For women aged 34 years or less, the chance of a live birth from one round of egg retrieval and IVF treatment was 52.4 per cent. For women aged between 35 and 44, however, there was a linear decline in the live birth rate. These figures are explained if you look at age and its relation to pregnancies per egg collection and miscarriages. For women aged between 34 and 37 there was a 39.2 per cent of a pregnancy per egg collection; 36.1 percent for 37 to 41 year olds; 21.8 per cent for 40 to 43 year olds; and a very low 5.4 per cent for 42 year olds.

Age and miscarriage were also related. Dr Jansen found that for women under 35 there was a 10.5 per cent chance of miscarriage per egg collection which rose to 16.1 per cent for women aged between 35 and 39 and to 42 per cent for those over 40.

Dr Jansen found that the most frequent users of IVF were women aged 39. However this was six years *after* the chances of success started to decline. He concluded his report by noting that: 'The community should be aware that, despite IVF, fertility ceases for an increasing proportion of women from their mid-thirties.'[17]

New directions in fertility treatment

The increasing use of IVF and related fertility treatments by older women has caused the industry to plough more research money into ways to trick Mother Nature, focusing on the nature and make-up of the egg and the culture medium in which the harvested embryos are kept. Pregnancy rates for older women have improved – according to IVF Australia pregnancy rates for women over 40 have doubled in the past five years. However as Dr Steven Steigrad noted in an article in 2004 about the success fertility groups are having impregnating older women, scientists still cannot stop some of these older women from miscarrying. 'Obviously when you hit 40, it's a very steep, slippery slope and until very recently we never had a woman over 42 conceive and keep the pregnancy.'[18]

Some of the leading research in fertility is being done in this area, which doesn't surprise Dr David Molloy, a Brisbane gynaecologist and specialist in infertility and reproductive medicine. He is also a clinical director of the Queensland Fertility Group (QFG). He says the number of older women coming to IVF is the greatest challenge facing reproductive technology.

It is a significant challenge for us and society as a whole. The fact that women have been delaying childbearing and are now paying the price by not being able to have children is a very important social trend. What role can IVF play in that trend? Well, it is a safety net. But that is all.

To make that net a little stronger, Dr Molloy and QFG are working on a new technique that targets the egg. The procedure is called mitochondrial transfer and injection, and QFG was the first clinic in Australia to use this procedure late in 2003. Dr Molloy says its aim is simple – to freshen up old eggs in women aged 37 and over. Mitochondria are the battery power packs of cells and in human eggs these packs can wear out. The new technique involves taking mitochondria from fresh cells and other parts of the woman's body and injecting them into her eggs. 'This basically provides a new power pack,' Dr Molloy says.

The procedure is still new – Taiwan is the only other country using it as part of fertility treatment. However, Dr Molloy is confident it will help boost an older woman's chances of falling pregnant from about 10 per cent to 40–45 per cent. He admits the focus of research has shifted because of the increasing demand from clients who have age-related infertility. He also admits there is only so much IVF can do.

The irony is that women find out too late that IVF and other fertility treatments can't help them. It is only when they are in their late thirties or forties and have tried and failed to have children that they find themselves at a fertility clinic where most of them hear the bad news for the first time.

So why do women wait?

It is taken for granted by many that women wait to have children because they want to establish their careers first. Many of the women interviewed for this book did just this. Manager Marian Hudson, editor Deborah Thomas and author/commentator Lisa Forrest were all busy building their professional lives during their twenties and thirties. Mind you, none of them were ruthless about having a career; their lives just seemed to carry them down this path, so that by the time they reached their late thirties they realised they had been too distracted by careers and life in general to focus on parenthood.

Kelly Hand, research officer with the Australian Institute of Family Studies noted in a paper she gave in 2001 titled, 'Supporting Older Mothers from Conception to Parenting', that the stereotype of older mothers as highly educated and career-focused is an accurate one. She quoted data from the Australian Family Project conducted in 1986 which showed a clear association between educational attainment and birth timing, with tertiary-educated women significantly more likely to delay the birth of their first child than other women.[19] Two studies by psychologists Julia Berryman and Kate Windridge in the United Kingdom also found that the older first-time mother was more likely to belong to non-manual and professional occupations.[20]

However, Hand is at pains to point out that identifying the pursuit of higher education and career as the sole reason why women delay starting families is contentious. There is the distraction factor we have just mentioned, when many women only find the time and space to focus on children when they reach their late thirties. And what about the concern women have about coping with work and family once the child is born? According to the Human Rights and Equal Opportunity Commission, increasing numbers of women put off having children because of work pressures and the expectation of women's primary role in childcare. Their website shows figures indicating a massive 54 per cent of women in one study believed that their careers had been affected by taking maternity leave. Forty-four per cent said their salaries stalled, 30.4 per cent believed their careers took a backward step and 29.9 per cent said they sacrificed their careers when they gave birth. The Commission concluded that low fertility rates indicated a growing trend by women to choose between work and family rather than seeking both.[21]

The mummy trigger

Many of the women I spoke to for this book talked about something triggering their desire to be a mother. It was an inexplicable feeling, a previously foreign maternal urge that made them desire to be a mother above all else. Not surprisingly, this urge intensifies when the desire is threatened.

This inexplicable feeling about motherhood has been examined by researchers and appears in a list of key life events and turning points that influence a woman's decision to have a child. Called the Six 'Ms' of Motherhood, they are:

- Mysterious metamorphosis, an unexplainable, insistent longing for a child.
- Menace of menopause, a fear that time is running out.
- Mortality; a reaction to the death of a parent, close friend or spouse.
- Money, the improvement or readjustment of personal finances.
- Maturity, the awareness of having matured and developed a stronger sense of self.
- Misplaced mothering, a determination to stop investing nurturing instincts in men.[22]

Research officer Kelly Hand, in her paper, concluded that research showed decision making about the timing of having children is a complex process. It can combine choices about career and self-development with what is seen as a twenty-first century necessity – the need to obtain a level of financial stability. Add to this the issues of circumstance, such as being in a relation-ship when the time is right.

Looking for Mr Right

Access to contraception and reproductive technology gives women more control over the timing of having children, meaning they can finish their education, often studying into their mid-twenties and then climb the career ladder before giving birth. Then there are older women who already have children but have remarried or are in a new relationship, and wish to start a family with their partner. But there is a subset of older women who are not voluntarily having late babies.

Maybe they have been forced to delay having children because of fertility problems that had not been solved into their late thirties even with the reproductive technology now avail-able. Or maybe they have always wanted children but failed to find the right partner. This can be just as crucial in the decision-making process as a woman's desire to find economic freedom through her education and career. It can affect a woman's belief that she can create enough security and love in her life to bring a child into the world. Anecdotal evidence of this isn't hard to find. How many times have you heard a woman in her thirties say she can't find a good man? Listen to Juanita Phillips's story of how she gave up on having children because she couldn't find a man who shared her commitment to having a family. Similarly a leading relationships counsellor told me of a forum she attended about family and work where, among the usual accusations about women being selfish because they waited until their thirties to have children and then expected special treatment in the workplace, there was one woman who stood up and said: 'Look I am tired of all this. Yes, I am 35 and I don't have children. Yes, I do have a career but if I had a partner I would change my priorities tomorrow.'

In 2003, Dr Veronica Clarke, a psychologist with Monash IVF in Melbourne, decided to find out why a growing number of women seeking fertility treatment were aged over 35. She wanted to understand their reasons for delaying childbearing and to ascertain women's expectations of their chances of achieving a live birth using ART.

She surveyed 152 clients. To be eligible to participate the women must not have had any previous IVF treatment, must be childless and had to be aged 35. They were asked what their reasons were for delaying childbearing until now. She gave them ten options to choose from, such as the need to pursue a career, the need to be financially secure or the need to meet family commitments.

She found that these reasons were influential, but over-whelmingly, the key reason given by women for delaying childbirth was because they were not in a suitable relationship.

This result did not surprise Dr Clarke.

What I had noticed in my clinical experience was that men were reluctant to commit. I think one of the reasons for this is the acceptability of cohabitation among young people. It has been transformed from something that was scandalous 25 to 30 years ago to something that is quite acceptable in its own right or as a prelude to marriage.

The second and third reasons for delaying childbearing were

the desire to pursue a career and the need to be financially secure. These results did not surprise Clarke either.

Some women, because of the enhanced educational and career opportunities available these days, choose to pursue careers or financial security. In our society it appears that we are indoctrinated into having this belief; that we are entitled to have it all, whatever the 'all' is. Subsequently, we want the house, and the car, the established career, and only then we believe we are ready to move on to having children.

Fair enough, but the second component of Dr Clarke's research revealed a potentially devastating combination. As part of her survey she also asked women how they rated their likelihood of a successful birth using IVF. In other words, were they realistic about their chances, given their age?

I found that 5 per cent were realistic about their chances. Most of them overestimated their chances. One of the survey participants was a medical doctor who was 42 and she rated her chances of success as more than 50 per cent, whereas in reality it can be as low as 10 per cent.

Dr Clarke would like gynaecologists and doctors to make women – and men – more aware of the negative impact of age on fertility.

What I get from my clinical experiences over and over again are women saying, 'Why didn't someone tell me this?' I think part of that is because in Western culture we have a very heavy reliance on science and technology. There are also the media head-lines about some famous 45-year-old's miracle baby. We do not talk about the heartbreak of so many other 45-year-olds.

America and the Netherlands have public campaigns, which inform women about the impact of age on their fertility. Such campaigns are needed in this country, something similar to the quit smoking campaigns. This is necessary so that for those women who choose to pursue a career or financial security, their decision is an informed one, which I do not believe is currently the case. Women still believe that because they are physically healthy, then whenever they are ready they can have a child.

Being informed about their reproductive ability may make women more aware of their reduced chances of having a baby later in life. But that doesn't change a key part of the equation when it comes to baby making, the importance of being in a relationship. In 2003, Ruth Weston, a research fellow at the Australian Institute of Family Studies agreed that relationships – or the lack of them – were a key point of interest.

I don't think enough has been made of relationships and their impact on fertility decision-making. Balancing work and family is important, but we also need to look at what happens when people float along in these cohabiting relationships which then break down.[23]

Women may also delay childbirth because they need to know they are financially secure. This is more acute in an era when many women are living away from extended family. Associate Professor Karen Thorpe maintains that a woman's need for emotional security can be vital in the decision to have children. Too often, she says, she reads media reports that take a simplistic approach to late babies. Career is often blamed for delayed motherhood; indeed on the day we speak there is a story in the newspaper about the record median age of mothers in Australia which simply cited career, then mortgage, as the reasons for older motherhood.[24]

Associate Professor Thorpe says twenty-first century society has put more focus on the need for a close partnership between a woman and a man before having children

We no longer have extended families around us as much as we used to; therefore we need other sorts of resources to support us in having children. Because this support network is very focused on just your partner these days, that is where the need for financial security is coming from.

He also says that studies in the United Kingdom have shown that often the sole support for women having a baby is their partner – hence the need to find a good one. Also, women without extended familial support frequently look to 'buy in' support, meaning they may wait until later in life when they have an established career and financial strength before trying to have children.

The fact that women think hard about what sort of partner they want before even considering children was also confirmed in a study in March 2004 by Monash University's Centre for Population and Urban Research. Titled *Men and Women Apart: The Decline of Partnering in Australia*, it found that women want guys with a degree of success. A good education and well-paid job greatly increased a man's chance of finding a mate however men with no tertiary qualifications were more likely to be single. The findings led the authors – Bob Birrell, Virginia Rapson and Clare Hourigan – to argue for a new focus in the debate on Australia's dwindling fertility rate. They said in their report: 'Though not denying the incentives to having children for women who find it difficult to combine paid work and motherhood, more attention should be placed on why men and women are not partnering and thus are not in a situation to begin contemplating having children.'[25]

Swing to singledom

In November 2003, the federal Employment and Workplace Relations Minister Kevin Andrews, in a report in *The Australian*, directly blamed the singles boom for Australia's stalled fertility rate. This swing to singledom was also noted in the Monash University study, *Men and Women Apart: The Decline of Partnering in Australia*, which reported that only a decade ago the great majority of young men and women aged 30–34 were married and so more likely to have established a secure relationship conducive to raising a family.

This is no longer the case. In 1986, 72 per cent of women aged 30–34 and 65 per cent of men aged 30–34 were married. By 2001, the comparable figures were 55 per cent for women and just 47 per cent for men.[26]

Just as it seems hard for men and women to find each other in the social maze that is the twenty-first century, it could be possible that young Australians are increasingly having trouble making the leap from fun relationship to real relationship in which children might be considered.

Dianne Gibson, national director of counselling at Relationships Australia, blames reality television shows such as *The Bachelor* for trivialising the art of forming a deep and meaningful relationship which has the strength to parent children.

> *How do you make this transition from going out to a singles bar and having great dates with someone into this other relationship which involves love and companionship? So what are the opportunities for really great women who are competent in their work lives to go out and meet someone? Where do they go to meet the comparable men? The old mechanisms which used to exist such as church fellowship, local clubs and sporting activities are gone. With so much focus away from communities and into work life we are not as well connected. The whole idea of how in our community we pair up is really very tricky now and I don't think we are coming to terms with that at all.*

Home bodies

Finding Mr Right obviously plays a vital role in a woman's decision to have babies but there are other general social factors that affect the late baby puzzle. There is a growing social trend for young people to live at home until their mid-twenties, meaning they might be even older than that by the time they establish a long-term relationship or gain economic independence.

This may be due to economic factors such as the increasing cost of a university education and the associated HECS debt, as well as the rising cost of home ownership. In December 2003, federal Labor education spokesperson Senator Jenny Macklin said reforms to tertiary education funding meant that the basic university degree would cost more than $20,000. 'That's what our young people will be starting their working lives with – a debt of $20,000.'[27]

Research by the National Centre for Social and Economic Modelling has also revealed that Generation X, the generation born between 1965 and 1980 cites HECS debts and expensive housing as factors in deferring having children.[28] In 1989, 65 per cent of 25 to 39-year-olds had already acquired their first home – this has now dropped to 54 per cent with 1 in 5 Gen Xers under 30 still living with their parents.

This trend was noted by Immigration Minister Amanda Vanstone who, in 2003, ignored any hint of a relationship crisis among thirty-somethings, to suggest that Australia's low fertility level was because we are too materialistic. 'We are a very, very material country and the current generations want everything,' said Senator Vanstone.[29]

The desire to have the latest plasma television, she reasoned, was impacting on the fertility rate because the only way to give children more was to have fewer of them.

On how to reverse this trend in fertility, Amanda Vanstone was more circumspect. She is a fan of increased immigration for Australia. She also said that studies had shown that inducements such as the baby bonus and paid maternity leave do not necessarily translate into a higher fertility rate.

Baby boom or bust

Anne Summers, in her 2003 book, *The End of Equality*, clearly shows why the women who could most afford to have a baby are the least likely to do so. She notes that young women today think long and hard about having a baby and or even becoming mothers at all. They see the change babies would bring to their lives and how having children can erode their financial base. Economist Dr Bruce Chapman from the Australian National University is quoted in the book as calculating that a woman who has completed secondary education will forgo lifetime earnings after tax of around $160,000 less than a woman who does not have a child.[30]

'Why are women having fewer and fewer babies?' Summers asked in an article she wrote for the *Medical Journal of Australia (MJA)*.

The reasons are complicated but the answer is in some ways surprisingly simple. As a society we ask women to give up too much when they have children and we give them far too little in return. The pleasures of children are, in the pragmatic calculus now undertaken by most young Australian women, not compensated for by what they have to forgo. They are expected to give up their jobs or at least cut back on them often after having been given a hard time while they were pregnant. They can expect to suffer a significant loss in earnings from which, over a lifetime, they will never recover as they will rarely be able to return to the same level of work as before. Is it any wonder there is a baby bust?[31]

Summers makes many valid points but she forgets that women, no matter how illogical or financially unsound it may be, will continue to have children. It will continue to be a battle for many, but they will become mums, with or without a baby bonus or universal paid maternity leave. Also, who knows what the younger generation of women will do. Perhaps, after watching their mothers frantically trying to juggle career, family and a relationship, they might decide to find their own way; a middle path which means they can enjoy motherhood and a life outside the home in a job that brings them economic security and personal satisfaction. Let us hope governments will consider this path carefully and deliver more family-friendly policies.

True, the number of childless women in this country is growing. How often have we heard young women in their late twenties or early thirties look at an associate with children who is rushing to meet family and work deadlines and utter: 'Too hard – no babies for me.'

Nevertheless, the fact remains that among women in their early thirties, Australia is experiencing something of a baby boom.

It is not that women don't want to have babies. In fact, the opposite is true. They want to have babies but social and economic forces, as well as that sometimes elusive element, finding a loving relationship, are making them delay motherhood. As women, we are in a biological bind, with our bodies primed for baby making in our late teens and early twenties – also the crucial time to enjoy our freedom, climb the corporate ladder or extend our education. Talk about bad timing. The words of Quentin Bryce, mother and grandmother, formerly federal Sex Discrimination Commissioner and now Governor of Queensland, never rang truer: 'You can have it all, but you can't have it all at once.'[32]

How do I know . . .

. . . If I am fertile?

It is estimated that up to 60 per cent of couples will conceive after three menstrual cycles and that 85 per cent will conceive within a year. At 35, it is not unusual for women to have to wait a year or more to conceive. In the Leicester Motherhood project conducted in the United Kingdom, the time taken to conceive was under six months for the majority of women, but over a quarter of first-time mothers of 35 plus took longer than two years to conceive their firstborn.[1]

Women who are concerned that there may be a problem should consult their doctor well within a year.

The key to understanding your fertility is knowing when and if you are ovulating. Ovulation is the monthly release of an egg from your ovary and it is the only time during the month that you can get pregnant. This means you have a two to three-day window of opportunity for the sperm and egg to come together to form an embryo. A lot of women believe they are most fertile at the end of their period however this not the case. The most fertile time is when you ovulate, which is in the middle of your menstrual cycle.

You can purchase Ovulation Predictor Kits (OPKs) which measure the amount of luteinising hormone in your urine. The level rises 24 to 36 hours before ovulation. You should have sex the day or two before ovulation and the day of ovulation. Remember, OPKs only show when you are about to ovulate – they won't tell you if you have actually released an egg.

OPKs are available at chemists for about $55. One stick (there are five in a pack) is used for each test and you need to test every 12 to 24 hours around the time of ovulation to catch your hormone surge. Estrogen levels peak when you are ovulating. Kits could be problematic for women over 40 who have premature ovarian failure, and the kits are harder to use if you don't have a regular cycle.

Another test checks your saliva for salt content, which rises as your oestrogen rises. It looks like a lipstick but is actually a tube fitted with a tiny lighted microscope and retails for about $80. You place your saliva on the lens, and as ovulation gets closer you should see a fern-shaped pattern. When the ferns cover the whole slide you are about to ovulate. This test can be reused and according to the US Food and Drug Administration is about 98 per cent accurate.

A more traditional method of checking ovulation is to take your temperature at the same time every morning before you get up and record the readings on a chart. You need to track a subtle drop in temperature followed by a sustained rise in temperature over three days. The drop occurs around ovulation and the rise indicates an increase in progesterone which occurs after you ovulate.

Research is also being done into ways in which women can test their ovarian reserves. This will help them know if they are going to encounter fertility problems in their thirties or forties. The research is being developed by Professor Robert Norman, head of the Reproductive Medicine Unit at Adelaide University. Late in 2003 he revealed he had trialled the tests on women undergoing IVF treatment. Blood tests measured hormones produced by the ovaries indicating the number and quality of eggs and ultrasound scans could pick up the number of developed eggs.[2]

For a deeper look at more diagnostic tests regarding fertility, look up Dr Robert Jansen's informative website, http://www.jansen.com.au/index.html

. . . How to boost fertility?

Okay, we can't beat Mother Nature and get a new batch of eggs at 40. However, we can change our lifestyle to boost our chances of conceiving. Here are some tips:

• Lose (or gain) weight. A woman who wishes to become pregnant should have a good diet and maintain at least an average body weight for her height. Research has shown that being overweight can have an impact on fertility – but so can being too thin. Being too thin could affect the regularity of menstrual cycles.

- Stop smoking. Smoking increases the risk of miscarriage and premature birth. It also has an adverse affect on the placenta which can be dangerous during pregnancy. Paternal smoking can also have an effect – one Finnish study showed that it could increase the risk of conception delay. Smoking can also bring on an earlier menopause in women.
- Reduce alcohol intake – preferably, don't drink at all.
- Consider the contraceptive pill. Research has shown that taking the pill for five years can extend your fertility. It also protects, or reduces, a lot of causes of infertility like pelvic inflammatory disease.
- Reduce stress. Easier said than done maybe, but exercise such as yoga or swimming is recommended to help de-stress.
- Revise your family history. Look into your family's reproductive history to see if there are any background fertility problems.
- Consult an expert. If you have any worries or doubts about fertility, see a gynaecologist or fertility expert.

Amanda Ellis's financial advice for new mothers

During my interviews with Amanda Ellis, economist at the World Bank, she talked passionately about how vital it is for women to be financially savvy and independent. This is especially important for women who are about to become mothers, and absolutely vital for older mothers who may not have the future earning power, because of their age, to stave off financial difficulties later in life.

The issue of how to protect yourself financially when you become a mother is critical for many women. When I thought about the financial pros and cons of having a child, from an economic point of view it made no sense to have a child. It has been estimated that the costs of the first child can be up to $160,000. Not having family-friendly policies, such as paid maternity leave, can make having a child even more expensive. Having *universal paid maternity leave would make it easier for many women and it has been proven that it saves organisations money as well. Westpac did a study and it showed that it saved up to $6 million a year by providing paid maternity leave because it did not have to spend money retraining and rehiring staff.*

So here's Amanda's advice on how to strengthen your finances and protect yourself as a new mum:

- Know your legal position at work. According to the Human Rights and Equal Opportunity Commission, an employee is generally entitled to return to the position she held prior to commencing leave or to a comparable position if her original job has ceased to exist. Employers should note that an employee may wish to return to work on a part-time basis, and some state laws specifically allow for return to work part-time after maternity leave by agreement with the employer. In some situations, an employer may be deemed to have discriminated if a reasonable request for part-time work is refused.

- If you are in an industry serviced by a union, make sure you touch base with your union when you go on maternity leave. This means you have someone to contact if there are problems when you return to work.

- If you want to have children, look for employers with family-friendly policies and practices. In other words, look at your employer and their attitude to maternity leave and part-time work. Is paid maternity leave available (only about 40 per cent of female employees in Australia are entitled to paid maternity leave), and how have other women in the workplace fared after they returned from maternity leave? Is there a positive attitude to new mothers returning from maternity leave and would you be offered some kind of part-time work if you wanted it?

- The smartest thing a woman can do is to ramp up her superannuation from an early age. Amanda's message is to start saving early. Australia's superannuation is largely an individual system where you only take out what you or your employer have put in. Therefore, when a woman is not earning funds are not going into her superannuation.

> *Unfortunately because a lot of women in Australia do not get paid maternity leave, any time that they are out of the workforce and not earning an income they are also not contributing to their superannuation. This is a real double whammy. The fact that women spend eighteen to twenty years in the workforce and men spend roughly double that, it is not surprising that women have only one-third of the retirement and superannuation savings compared to men. Yet women have a longer lifespan then men. So what we have is a huge problem with older women who are living in poverty.*

- As well as saving from an early age into a superannuation fund, it is beneficial to budget.

> *I know it sounds boring and everyone hates to think of doing a budget, but it works. We have a spreadsheet in our computer at home and we know what all our major expenses are each month and we track these. I suggest that people start to work out where their major expenditure is and then decide what can be cut and what is non-negotiable.*

It is all about working out your own money personality so you can see where you can cut back in a way that won't be as painful when you have had the baby. It's hard enough worrying about the baby without worrying about your finances at this time as well.

Endnotes

Maggie Alderson

1. Jackie Meyers-Thompson and Sharon Perkins, *Fertility for Dummies*, Wiley, New York, 2003.

Juanita Phillips

1. Gil Chalmers, 'Juanita's whirlwind romance', *Australian Women's Weekly*, July 2003.
2. George Megalogenis, *Faultlines: Race, Work and the Politics of Changing Australia*, Scribe Publications, Melbourne, 2003.

Alannah Hill

1. Kate Halfpenny, 'Flower child', *Who*, 20 October 2003, p. 128.

Deborah Thomas

1. Nancy Gibbs, 'Making time for baby', *Time*, 15 April 2002, p. 47.

Lisa Forrest

1. Sue Williams, 'Lisa Forrest's labour of love', *Australian Women's Weekly*, July 2003, p. 44.

Marian Hudson

1. Susan Faludi, *Backlash: The Undeclared War Against Women*, Chatto & Windus, London, 1991, pp. 46–47.
2. Ruth Pollard, 'Pregnant pause that will leave 71ers childless forever', *Sydney Morning Herald*, 5 February 2003, p. 4.

Jacki MacDonald

1. Ronnie Gibson, 'Exit wacky Jacki with a tearful quip', *Sunday Mail*, 28 May 1989, p. 3.
2. Paul Wicks, 'Wacky Jacki to start a family', *Courier-Mail*, 25 May 1989, p. 1.
3. Kerrie Theobald, 'New baby, new career', *Australian Women's Weekly*, August 1995, p. 28.

Lisa Bolte

1. Valerie Lawson, 'Bolte's final pas de deux as mother's role beckons', *Sydney Morning Herald*, 27 April 2002, p. 2.

Claudia Keech

1. Mercedes Florez, 'Men who sacrifice for love: why some husbands are putting their partner's career first', *Sunday Telegraph*, 23 December 2001, p. 28.
2. Rachel Browne, 'Late expectations: Time waits for no mum, even Elle Macpherson', *Sun-Herald*, 18 August 2002, p. 48.
3. 2003 Relationships Indicator Survey, Relationships Australia, Relationships Australia National, Canberra, 2003.

Amanda Ellis

1. Nancy Gibbs, 'Making time for baby', *Time*, 15 April 2002, p. 47.

Mary-Rose MacColl

1. Debra Aldred, 'Stranger of the family', *Courier-Mail*, 12 April 2003, p. 3.

The trend to older motherhood

1. 'Age of women giving birth now older than ever', *Births, Australia 2002*, Australian Bureau of Statistics (Cat. no. 3301.0), Canberra, 2002, p. 12.
2. *Births, Australia 2002*, Australian Bureau of Statistics, ibid, p. 6.
3. *Australian Social Trends 2002: Population – Population Projections: Fertility Futures*, Australian Bureau of Statistics (Cat. no. 4102.0), Canberra, 2002, p. 12.
4. *Australian Social Trends 2002*, Australian Bureau of Statistics, ibid, p. 37.
5. *Australian Social Trends 2002*, Australian Bureau of Statistics, ibid, p. 12.
6. David De Vaus, *Fertility Decline in Australia*, Australian Institute of Family Studies, Family Matters, no. 63, 2002, p. 14.
7. David De Vaus, ibid, p. 21.
8. Julia Berryman, Karen Thorpe and Kate Windridge, *Older Mothers: Conception, Pregnancy and Birth after 35*, Pandora, London, 1995, p. 108.
9. Nancy Gibbs, 'Making time for baby', *Time*, 15 April 2002, p. 47.
10. Sylvia Ann Hewlett, *Baby Hunger: The New Battle for Motherhood*, Atlantic Books, London, 2002, p. 93.
11. Nancy Gibbs, 'Making time for baby', *Time*, ibid.
12. Berryman et al., *Older Mothers*, p. 106.
13. Deborah Smith, 'Endless supply of eggs raises fertility hopes for women', *Sydney Morning Herald*, 12 March 2004, p. 1.
14. Nancy Gibbs, 'Making time for baby', *Time*, p. 47.

15. Zoe Taylor, 'Body clock alarm, women misled on fertility', *Daily Telegraph*, 12 November 2003, p. 9.

16. IVF Australia website, IVF Australia: www.ivf.com.au

17. Robert Jansen, 'The effect of female age on the likelihood of a live birth from one in-vitro fertilisation treatment', *Medical Journal of Australia*, vol. 178, 17 March 2003, p. 261.

18. Miranda Wood, 'IVF Success rates rise as technology kicks in', *Sun-Herald*, 4 April 2004, p. 12.

19. Kelly Hand, 'Supporting older mothers from conception to parenting', paper presented at one-day forum for Tweddle Child and Family Health Service and Victoria University (nursing), Victoria University, 27 July 2001, p. 3.

20. Berryman et al., *Older Mothers*, p. 30.

21. Website, Human Rights & Equal Opportunity Commission: www.hreoc.gov.au

22. Schlesinger & Scheslinger, 'Postponed parenthood: trends and issues', *Journal of Comparative Family Studies*, vol. 29, no. 3, Autumn, 1989, pp. 353–363.

23. Christine Jackman and Ann Clark, 'And mother makes two', *The Australian*, 10–11 May 2003, p. 19.

24. Tanya Moore, 'Median age of first-time mothers at record high', *Courier-Mail*, 19 November 2003, p. 3.

25. Bob Birrell, Virginia Rapson, Clare Hourigan, *Men and Women Apart: The Decline of Partnering in Australia*, Centre for Population and Urban Research, Monash University, Melbourne, April 2004, p. 9.

26. Birrell et al., ibid.

27. Malcolm Cole, 'Debts to weigh on undergraduates', *Courier-Mail*, 6 December 2003, p. 4.

28. Monica Videnieks and Caitlin Fitzsimmons, 'Boomers beware wrath of Gen Xcluded', *The Australian*, 18 November 2003, p. 2.

29. Cynthia Banham, Jeff Fleischer and Mark Coultan, 'Why we've got to get back to the clucky country', *Sydney Morning Herald*, 2 December 2003, p. 1.

30. Anne Summers, *The End of Equality: Work, Babies and Women's choices in Twenty-first Century Australia*, Random House, Sydney, 2003, p. 159.

31. Anne Summers, 'The Baby Bust', *Medical Journal of Australia*, no. 178, 2002, p. 612.

32. Amanda Ellis, *Women's Business, Women's Health*, Random House, Sydney, 2002, p. 352.

How do I know . . .

1. Julia Berryman, Karen Thorpe and Kate Windridge, *Older Mothers: Conception, pregnancy and birth after 35*, HarperCollins, London, 1995. p. 71.

2. Judy Skatssoon, 'Infertility test to help families plan babies', *Courier-Mail*, 12 November 2003, p. 16.

Abbreviations

ABS – Australian Bureau of Statistics
ART – Assisted Reproductive Technology
CVS – Chorionic villus sampling
IVF – In-vitro fertilisation
OECD – Organization for Economic Cooperation and
Development

Glossary

Amniocentesis: An amniocentesis involves taking a small sample of amniotic fluid (water) from around the developing foetus. A needle is first passed through the pregnant woman's skin, then through the wall of the uterus (womb), and on the amniotic fluid. An amniocentesis is offered to women of 37 years and over at the estimated time of delivery. It is usually done from 14–16 weeks and is used to detect chromosome abnormalities such as Down syndrome, Neural tube defects (ie spina bifida or anencephaly), and some inherited disorders in those couples who have been shown to be at high risk, eg cystic fibrosis.

Chorionic villus sampling (CVS): A test done at 10 or 12 weeks in which a needle is passed into the developing placenta. A few small fragments of the tissue are drawn up into a syringe. Tests on the tissue can show if the developing foetus has certain abnormalities. It is also known as placenta biopsy or placentocentesis.

CVS is offered to women who will be 37 years or over when they give birth.

Clomid: An estrogen-like drug used to induce ovulation. Also known as Clomoiphene citrate. Clomid acts by causing a gland in the brain to release hormones which stimulate ovulation.

Down syndrome: A chromosomal disorder caused by an error in cell division which in its most common form produces an additional third chromosome 21 or trisomy 21. The abnormality can result in mental retardation and certain physical characteristics such as slanting eyes and 'floppy' muscle tone.

In-vitro fertilisation (IVF): When fertilisation – the moment when the egg and sperm join – takes place in a test tube rather than in the womb. The resulting embryo is then implanted in the uterus.

Primigravida: A woman who is having her first pregnancy.

Primiparae: A woman who is giving birth for the first time.

Did you know?

- Late babies are those born to women over 35 years of age. These women are termed 'elderly primigravida' or 'elderly primiparae'.
- The average age of first-time mothers is increasing. In 2002, the median age of Australian mothers was 30.2 – the highest on record.
- Women aged 35–39 have more than doubled their rate of giving birth since 1982. However, fertility rates for women aged 29 have halved over the past two decades.
- The average age of fathers is increasing, with first-time dads most likely to be aged 32.5 years.
- In 2002 Australia's fertility rate was 1.75 babies per woman – half the 1961 figure when fertility rates peaked at 3.5 babies per woman.
- According to 2000 estimates, about 25 per cent of women

currently in their reproductive years will remain childless.

- Women are most fertile between the ages of 18 and 27. Fertility starts to decline from 27, with the decrease accelerating into a woman's thirties and early forties.

- At a woman's most fertile peak she has a 25 per cent chance of falling pregnant in a menstrual cycle.

- By the time a woman reaches 40, she has only a 5 per cent chance each cycle. This compares to about 20 per cent for a woman in her early thirties and 10–15 per cent for a woman aged 35–40.

- IVF is the most popular form of assisted conception. However, experts warn that its success rate varies considerably and it is not a solution to age-related infertilty. For women aged between 22 and 34 there is a 50.4 per cent success rate using IVF. This rate plummets to just 15 per cent for women aged between 39 and 44 years.

- The risks of miscarriage and chromosomal abnormalities in the foetus are higher for women in their late thirties and early forties. A 20-year-old woman has a 1 in 1340 chance of having a baby with Down syndrome. This risk leaps to 1 in 60 for a 42-year-old woman.

Recommended reading

Julia Berryman, Karen Thorpe and Kate Windrige, *Older Mothers: Conception, Pregnancy and Birth After 35*, Pandora, London, 1995.

Kaz Cooke, *Up the Duff*, Viking/Penguin, Melbourne, 2002.

Rachel Cusk, *A Life's Work: On Becoming a Mother*, Fourth Estate, London, 2001.

Amanda Ellis, *Women's Business, Women's Health: Create the Life You Want at Work and in Business*, Random House, Sydney, 2002.

Susan Faludi, *Backlash: The Undeclared War Against Women*, Chatto & Windus, London, 1991.

Sylvia Ann Hewlett, *Baby Hunger: The New Battle for Motherhood*, Atlantic Books, London, 2002.

Sheila Kitzinger, *Birth Over 35*, Sheldon Press, London, 1994.

Jean Liedloff, *The Contiuum Concept*, Arkana/Penguin, London, 1986.

Jackie Meyers-Thompson & Sharon Perkins, *Fertility for Dummies*, Wiley, New York, 2003.

Sarah Napthali, *Buddhism for Mothers: A Calm Approach To Caring For Yourself and Your Children*, Allen & Unwin, Sydney, 2003.

Anne Summers, *The End of Equality: Work, Babies and Women's Choices in Twenty-first Century Australia*, Random House, Sydney, 2003.

Deborah J. Swiss & Judith Walker, *Women and the Work-Family Dilemma: How Today's Professional Women Are Confronting the Maternal Wall*, John Wiley & Sons, Toronto, 1993.

Gil Thorn, *Not too Late: Having a Baby After 35*, Bantam, London, 1998.

Naomi Wolf, *Misconceptions*, Vintage, London, 2001.

Websites

Wellwomen's Website: www.rwh.org.au

IVF Australia: www.ivf.com.au

The Fertility Society of Australia: www.fsa.au.com

Mothers 35 plus: www.oldermothers.co.uk

ITA, Infertility Treatment Authority: www.ita.org.au

Melbourne IVF: www.mivf.edu.au

Monash IVF: www.monashivf.edu.au

Queensland Fertility Group: www.qldfertilitygroup.com.au

Bubhub: www.bubhub.com.au

MothersInc: www.mothersinc.com.au

Dr Robert Jansen: www.jansen.com.au

Acknowledgements

Writing a book like this would have been impossible without the honesty and faith of the women who were interviewed. A heartfelt thanks to all twelve women, all of them busy people, who devoted precious time to tell me their stories about the late babies in their lives. Their candour and willingness to be frank and open about their experiences made me all the more determined to write the book.

Late Babies would not have happened without time – time to do the interviews, the research and to write. This would not have been possible without the support of The Courier-Mail's editor, David Fagan, and features editor, Brian Crisp, who, at short notice, agreed to let me take long-service leave.

Nor would it have survived without the passion and insight of the women at Random House who embraced the idea for this book right from the start and never let go. So, many thanks to

Carol Davidson, Jane Southward, Katie Stackhouse and freelance editor Amanda O'Connell.

Help also came from other quarters and I am very grateful to my friend Alison Walsh for reading the book in between trying to manage her own busy life with work and twin boys. I'm grateful also to Justine Walpole for patiently taking photos of myself and son Hamish.

Finally, I need to acknowledge my very own ideas man, my husband Phil Brown. It was his idea to write a book about having a baby late in life. Once the idea was hatched he encouraged and inspired me to go on, making tea at the right moments and taking Hamish for some very, very long outings.

About the author

Sandra McLean has been a journalist for 23 years, starting her career as a cadet on the *Sunday Sun* newspaper in Brisbane. In 1985, after graduating with a degree in journalism from the University of Queensland, and having spent four years on a tabloid newspaper doing everything from death knocks to restaurant reviews, she embarked on a magical mystery tour of South-East Asia, Nepal and Europe, arriving in London in 1986 to work for News Ltd and the American wire service, United Press International. Since then she has worked in Australia as a freelance writer, sub-editor and section editor for newspapers and magazines such as the *Sunday Mail* in Brisbane and *TV Week* in Melbourne. In 1997 she was appointed Arts Editor of the *Courier-Mail*, a position she held for four years before taking maternity leave in mid-2000 to have her son, Hamish, at the age of 38. After a year off, she returned to the *Courier-Mail* where she is now a senior feature writer. She lives in the Brisbane suburb of Wilston with her husband, Phil Brown, who is also a journalist (and a poet/surfer/author) and Hamish, 4.